NATURAL
HOME PHARMACY

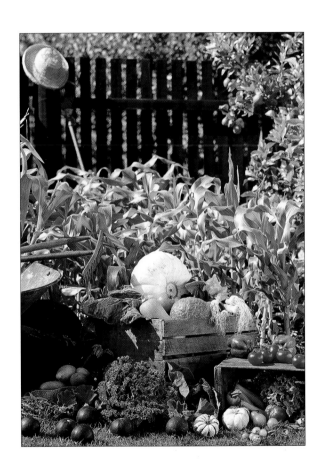

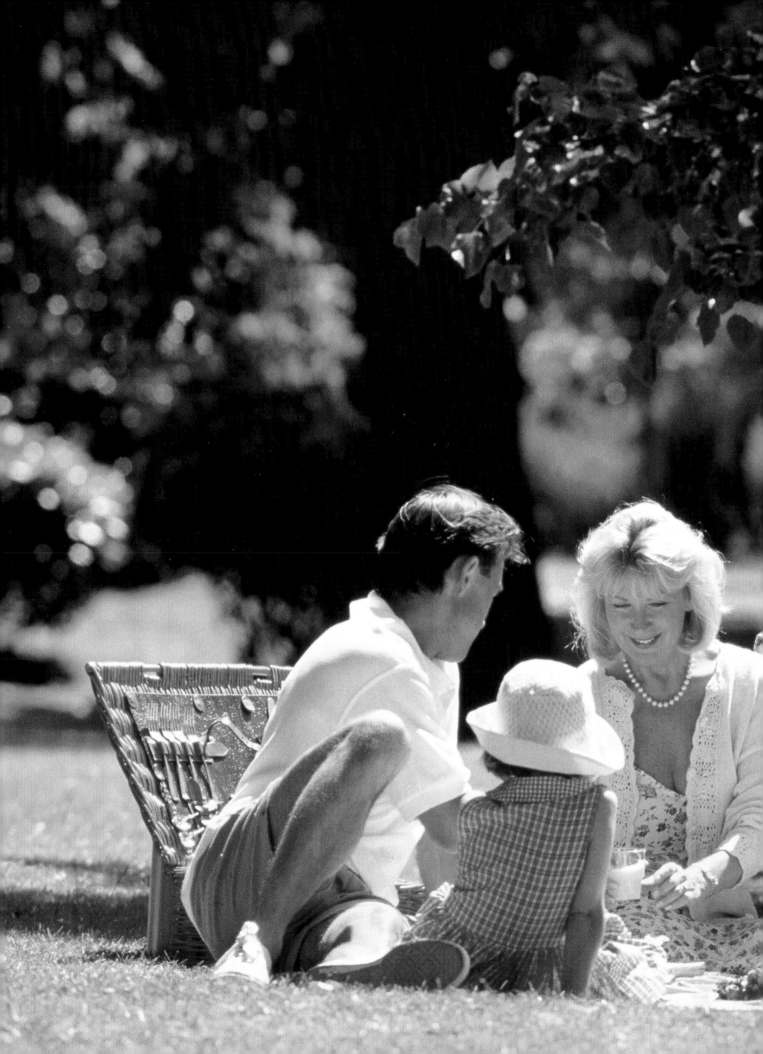

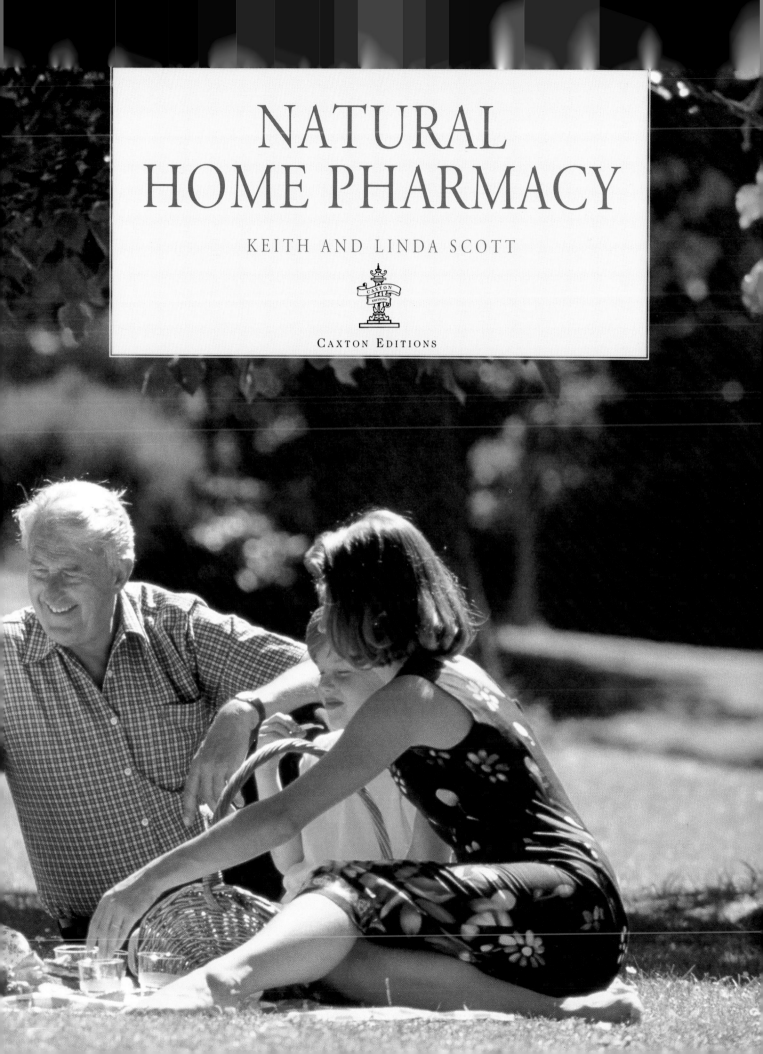

NATURAL
HOME PHARMACY

KEITH AND LINDA SCOTT

CAXTON EDITIONS

This edition published 2002 by Caxton Editions
an imprint of The Caxton Publishing Group

First published in the UK in 1998 by
New Holland Publishers (UK) Ltd
London • Cape Town • Sydney • Auckland

10 9 8 7 6

ISBN 1 84067 339 7

Senior Designer: Lyndall du Toit
Concept Design: Petal Palmer
Editors: Sally Rutherford and Laura Milton
Project Manager: Linda de Villiers
Picture Researcher: Carmen Swanepoel
Illustrators: Philippa Allen, Steven Felmore,
Christine Hart-Davies, Georgina Steyn
Stylist: Marjo Kranenborg
Indexer: Sandie Vahl

Reproduction by cmyk Pre-press (Pty) Ltd
Printed and bound by Times Offset (M) Sdn. Bhd.

Photographic credits
All photographs except for those listed below were taken by Craig Fraser for the Struik Image Library.
M. Alexander, pp. 113 (top right), 114 (right); Michael D. Bryan/Photo Access, p. 19; Jim Cummins/Photo Access, p. 51;
Paolo Curto/The Image Bank, p. 24; John Cutten/Mary Evans Picture Library, p. 64; Georgette Douwma/Photo Access/
Planet Earth Pictures, p. 101 (top); Focal Point Photo Library, pp. 56/57; J.P. Fruchet/Photo Access, pp. 78/79;
Tipp Howell/Photo Access/V.C.L., pp. 123, 136; Kim Hutton/ABPL, p. 18 (top); Instant Images, (authors' picture, dust
jacket back flap); Jeff Kaufman/Photo Access, p. 25; Udo Kroner/All Over Bild Archiv, p. 61; Bill Ling/Photo Access, pp. 2/3;
Bill Losh/Photo Access, p. 127; Jay Matthews/Landmarks, p. 131; Daniel Pangbourne/Photo Access, p. 21; Uwe Schmid/
All Over Bild Archiv, p. 80; Superstock Photography (Breughel), p. 86; Arthur Tilley/Photo Access, p. 95 (top right);
Lisa Trocchi/SIL, p. 96; Mel Yates/Photo Access, pp. 50, 65 (top).

Illustrators' credits
Philippa Allen/SIL, pp. 12, 15, 24, 32, 46, 50, 58, 64, 66/67, 70 (top), 74, 80, 83, 85;
Steven Felmore/SIL, pp. 70 (bottom), 72 (top, middle, bottom), 73 (left and right), 75 (top right), 76 (top
right), 77 (bottom), 94, 97, 98, 99 (top right), 102, 107, 110, 113, 115, 117, 118, 119, 122, 124, 125, 126;
Christine Hart-Davies/New Holland Publishers, all herb drawings from pages 37 to 45 except for those listed
below, drawn by Georgina Steyn/SIL, pp. 37 (Huang Qi and Rooibos), 38 (Green/Black Tea and Hawthorne),
41 (Californian Poppy, Siberian Ginseng and Maidenhair Tree), 42 (Saw Palmetto and Milk Thistle),
45 (Chaste Tree/Agnus Castus, Bilberry and Guelder Rose/Cramp Bark), 99 (bottom left), 128 (bottom left).

AUTHORS' ACKNOWLEDGEMENTS

We would like to thank the following people who helped in many different ways with our communication problems: Joe Beale of Abacus Computers, Selebi-Phikwe; Louis-John and Matie Botha; Chris Scholtz of Ellisras Pharmacy and last, but not least, Lyn Nevill and Frank Jones of Phikwe Industrial Metal Pressing.

For entrusting us with the project our thanks go to Linda de Villiers.

For making the project a reality thanks to Sally Rutherford and Laura Milton (who had to take over in the final stages) for their incisive editorial work and patience with our many changes; Lyndall du Toit for her inspired design work; Craig Fraser for his wonderful photographs and willingness to stretch his limits and Marjo Kranenborg who doubled as a stylist and stunning model. To the other models, Elmori Richter, Beverley Dodd, Paul Matthews, Linda Fielding and baby James Negus, we extend our gratitude for your part in the beautiful photographs that illustrate this book. The photo shoots were an experience to be fondly remembered.

We would also like to thank Sally and Rawdon Ball for their open door policy and support; Sandi and Peter Unite for their hospitality and the use of their wonderful beach house; Lorraine Forbes for helping to get the project started; Jean Kiekopf for her support; Robyn and Charles Sheldon for their hospitality and willingness to share a new direction, and Linda's parents, Joan and Terry McCourt and sister, Karen Coetzee for their support and hospitality during extended working holidays in Cape Town. Our final thanks go to our three children, Robyn, Damien and Lauren, who have been, in more ways than one, a big part of this book.

IMPORTANT NOTICE

The advice and treatment instructions contained in this book are of a general nature and are not specific to any individual's particular requirements. It is imperative, therefore, not to attempt self-treatment of serious or undiagnosed long-term complaints. If your condition fails to improve, professional advice must be sought. Also seek professional advice before undertaking any self-treatment while undergoing prescribed medical treatment. Many treatments can cause allergic or adverse reactions in very sensitive individuals. If this happens, discontinue the treatment immediately and seek professional help if the symptoms do not abate.

The authors and publishers, while both hoping that the advice given here will be of a beneficial nature, cannot accept responsibility for any adverse reactions to the treatment suggestions.

CONTENTS

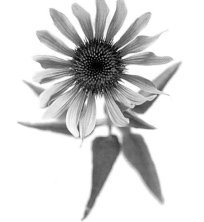
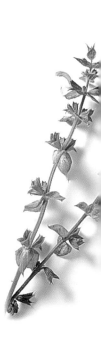
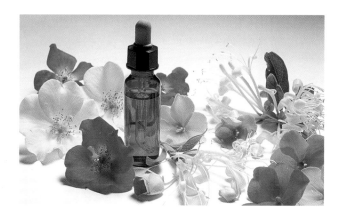

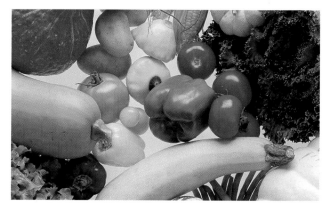

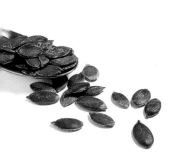

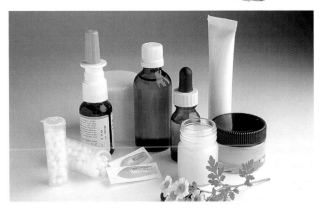

AILMENT AND TREATMENT
GLOSSARY 88

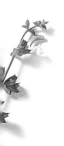

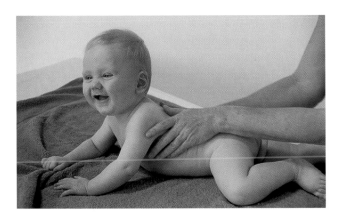

FOREWORD

Linda and Keith Scott have spent many years researching and studying the subject of complementary therapies. This book is a testament to their success. It is an informative and easy-to-use guide which explains the 'why' as well as the 'how'. Keith's medical background has ensured that safety of use is paramount, and throughout, readers are reminded that if they are unsure, if symptoms deteriorate or if no change occurs over time, they should consult a qualified practitioner. This sensible and practical book allows the reader to understand the essentials of health and the prevention of 'dis-ease' as well as guiding them in the direction of self-help.

Each part of *Natural Home Pharmacy* is introduced with a basic, easy-to-understand section which leads into the self-help treatment guide. The vital importance of nutrition, exercise and the mind/body interaction are explored before the reader is taken forward to treat symptoms. This is an unusual but hugely refreshing aspect of the book. By encouraging health, Linda and Keith are saying prevention is better than cure. This extremely positive approach to wellbeing is a central theme of naturopathy and the other complementary disciplines, but is only recently becoming part of the medical approach.

The self-help directory is well presented and is full of good, sensible advice. The basic premise – that health comes from within – remains, and this is built upon using external and topical applications to aid the self-reparative and self-restorative abilities of the body. These methods are outlined for each condition, with a range of nutritional, herbal, homeopathic, supplemental, aromatherapeutic, Bach and other remedies. With each presenting problem a short description allowing the patient to focus more accurately on the condition is followed by general dietary advice plus specific remedies. Each condition is supported, where appropriate, by clear explanatory diagrams or illustrations allowing the patient to localize points accurately. Each treatment is clear and easy to follow with, where indicated, a special precautionary or warning note. Throughout, safety is paramount and advice is given to seek qualified help if in doubt.

This well-written, well-presented and informative book will be an asset to any home reference shelf while most practitioners will come to value it as a positive addition to their own reference collection and a reliable source of advice for patients seeking self-help.

DR IAN DRYSDALE BSc (Hons), PhD (Lond), ND, DO
PRINCIPAL OF THE BRITISH COLLEGE OF NATUROPATHY AND OSTEOPATHY

INTRODUCTION

In 1976 Keith was a newly qualified doctor, working for the National Health Service in Britain when, with his fresh enthusiasm, he believed that most diseases could be cured or controlled with drugs, radiation or surgery. I was a student at Oxford who, like most of my contemporaries, saw illness as an irritation that was more or less in the hands of fate. If you fell ill you simply went to a doctor who cured you with drugs. We were both fortunate, however, to meet a doctor, David Jenkins, who questioned both beliefs and the direction modern medicine was taking. He saw that, in spite of a massive increase in drug prescriptions and surgery, the incidence of chronic disease had increased by 50 percent in the last couple of decades.

Over huge bean feasts cooked on bunsen burners in the Oxford University physiology laboratory, he convinced us that we were largely responsible for our own diseases. He showed us research implicating diets which were high in refined foods and low in fibre (a typical Western diet), in the development of appendicitis, diverticulitis, cancer of the colon, high cholesterol levels and diabetes. We became enthusiastic converts to this way of thinking and spent the next twenty years investigating other ways in which we could safely – yet effectively – control our own health, without recourse to drugs and surgery. Our three children became unwitting co-investigators, as did our friends and Keith's many patients – first in South Africa, then England and New Zealand, followed currently by those in Botswana. We can now say with confidence that everything we eat, drink, feel, think and do are all important factors in the equation of health.

Modern medicine has reached a crossroads. While it has many areas of excellence in the field of infectious diseases, vaccinations and orthopedic and reconstructive surgery, it has many areas of weakness, especially concerning chronic degenerative diseases and psychiatric problems. These problems, coupled with growing concern over antibiotic-resistant bacteria and an increasing incidence of iatrogenic diseases (those caused by medical treatment), has led to a substantial defection away from orthodox medicine of not only patients, but doctors as well.

1n 1985 one out of five people in England consulted a complementary practitioner – today that figure is closer to one out of three. Many doctors have now incorporated complementary therapies into their practices or happily refer their patients to such practitioners. The same trend appears to be happening in other developed countries. A revolution is underway.

This book is not definitive, but represents a distillation of our collective practical experience. It has been written to help people who want to join in by starting to take as much responsibility as possible for their own health and mental wellbeing. We wish you success.

Linda Scott

LINDA SCOTT
MA (Oxon)

Keith Scott

DR KEITH SCOTT
MB ChB (Cape Town), MF Hom (UK)

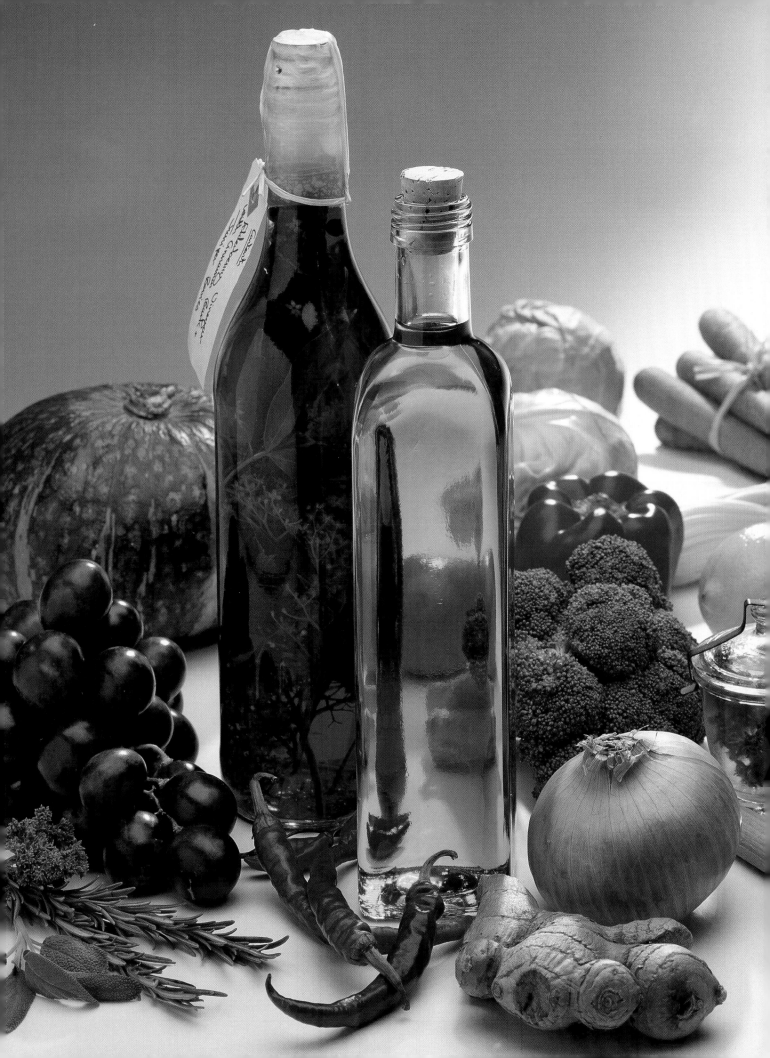

NATURE'S REMEDIES AND THERAPIES

*T*he types of food we eat and the way we exercise our bodies both have far-reaching implications for our physical and mental health. Nature's pharmacy is abundantly stocked with foods and herbs that can help protect us from physical disease and mental disharmony. Plant foods, including herbs, offer the most protection. In addition to vitamins and minerals, that are also present in animal foods, plants come packed full of other factors that prevent disease. These include dietary fibre, carotenoids, bioflavonoids, phytosterols, phytoestrogens and various other phytonutrients. This chapter explains which foods are harmful, how to use foods, herbs and aromatic oils to heal and prevent disease, why supplements are often necessary and how exercise can promote a healthier mind and body.

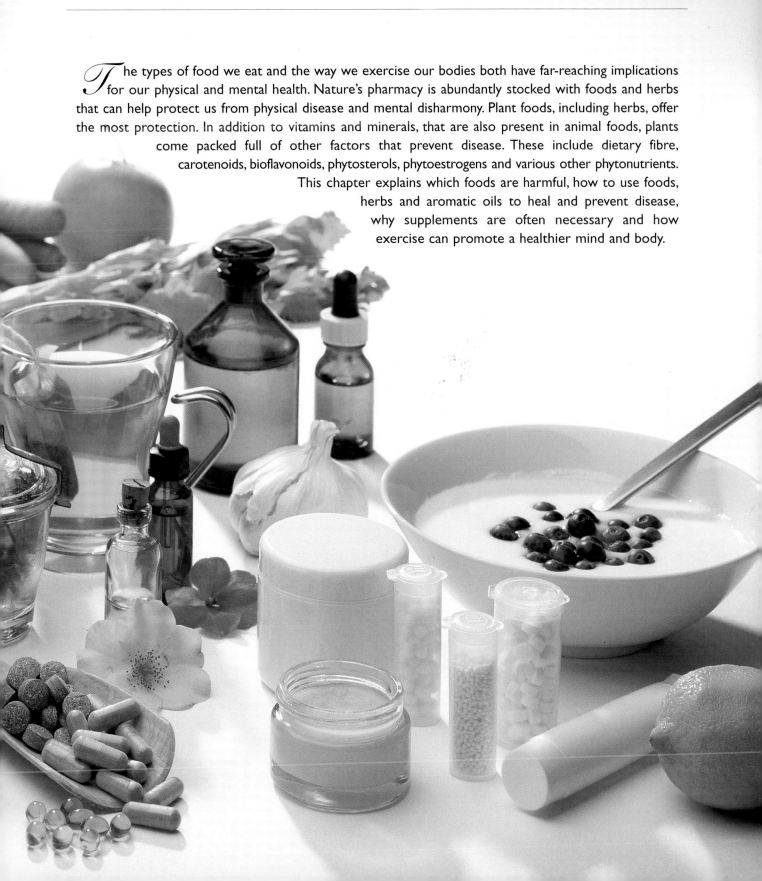

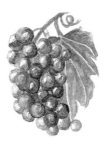

EATING FOR HEALTH

People living in the developed world have unwittingly participated in the largest uncontrolled trial ever undertaken by humans. The experiment is not over, but the results are already conclusive: eating a diet radically different from that which predominated during our evolutionary development has serious health consequences. Cardiovascular disease, strokes, hypertension, diabetes, obesity, gout, appendicitis, allergies, chronic degenerative diseases and mental illness are all directly associated with a typical Western diet. The main causes are too much animal fat, sugar, salt and alcohol, too many refined grains, processed foods and food additives, too little fibre, fruit and vegetables, and modern farming methods which rely heavily on chemicals and artificial fertilizers.

An understanding of how certain foods benefit or harm us offers us the single most important way of controlling our health and sense of wellbeing. While foods contain the nutrients that are essential for life, such as amino acids, carbohydrates, essential fatty acids, vitamins and minerals, they are not simply vehicles for these nutrients. Each food-type comes with a diverse array of extra substances which have far-reaching effects on every biological process in the body.

Although well-established dietary guidelines exist for promoting and maintaining health, there are exceptions. People are unique: not everyone eating a high salt diet will develop hypertension, nor will everyone overloading with sugar develop diabetes. On the other hand, those with a gluten intolerance (estimated to be one person in 250) will develop severe absorption problems if they eat any 'healthy' wholegrain foods containing gluten (wheat, rye, barley and oats). There is no such thing as a healthy diet for one and all: one person's meat can certainly be another's poison! Nevertheless, the basic guidelines for healthy eating should be followed. (If following the basic guidelines is a radical departure from your usual diet, you may experience temporary side-effects including headaches, abdominal discomfort and lethargy; if these persist they may indicate a food allergy.)

BASIC GUIDELINES FOR HEALTHY EATING

- Ensure a good intake of fresh vegetables and fruit. Vegetables, especially the green leafy variety, (5 servings daily) and fruit (2–4 servings daily) should dominate the diet. As many minerals, vitamins and other nutrients are destroyed by heat or lost in the cooking water as much food as possible should be eaten raw. The rest should be lightly steamed, baked, microwaved or added to stews.
- Eat sufficient dietary fibre in the form of pulses, brown rice, oats, barley, corn, seeds, nuts and wholemeal bread (3–4 servings daily).
- Cut down on foods with a high saturated fat content, such as meat, poultry and dairy products.
- Eliminate all artificially saturated fats such as margarine and vegetable shortening. Fats should comprise less than 30% of your total energy intake. In an 8 400 kJ (2 000 calorie) diet, this means you should eat less than 67 grams (2½ oz) of fat daily, two-thirds of which should be unsaturated.
- Eat fish such as mackerel, trout, tuna and salmon, which are rich sources of the important omega 3 fatty acids. If you cannot tolerate fish, take a daily supplement of 1 tbsp flaxseed oil.
- Intake of refined carbohydrates (white bread, pastry and so on) and sweet foods and drinks should be minimal and reserved for special occasions. Contrary to popular belief, sugar is not an essential nutrient and its high intake in the West contributes to many diseases.
- Intake of salt, alcohol, tea and coffee should all be limited or excluded.
- Ready-prepared and processed foods should be avoided as they contain a multitude of additives which can cause a range of problems, from asthma to hyperactivity. Check food labels for additives and become a discriminating shopper.
- Drink at least six glasses of bottled or filtered water daily.

VEGETARIAN/VEGAN DIETS

If you choose to eat a vegetarian or vegan diet, it is important that you learn how to combine and balance the food you eat so that you receive the full nutritional requirements of your body. It is necessary to restructure your entire diet and way of eating to ensure that you receive the full range of required nutrients.

BALANCING YOUR DIET

This food pyramid shows which foods should predominate in the diet and which should be eaten more sparingly. Vegetarians and vegans should eat a daily selection of some of the foods listed in italics in the same proportions indicated by their position in the food pyramid. Everyone should eat a wide variety of foods.

FATS
olive oil,
butter, cheese

PROTEINS
nuts, seeds, soya-based products,
skinless poultry, lean meat, low-fat
dairy products, eggs, fish

COMPLEX CARBOHYDRATES
rice, wholewheat products (pasta and bread), millet,
corn, oats, rye, barley (or any wholegrains)

PULSES, VEGETABLES AND FRUIT
peas, beans (adzuki, kidney, pinto, haricot, black-eyed, lima, chickpeas), lentils, cabbage,
broccoli, leafy green vegetables, green peppers, brussels sprouts, potatoes, onions, carrots, squash,
tomatoes, sweet potatoes, citrus fruits, grapes, berries, apples, melons, apricots,
peaches, avocadoes, papaya, bananas, plums

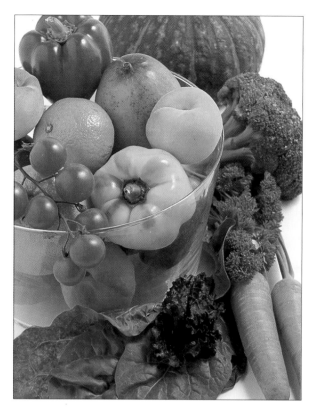

Above: *All yellow, orange and red fruits and vegetables contain carotenoids. Dark green vegetables such as broccoli and spinach are also excellent sources.*

Below: *Pulses are a valuable source of dietary fibre, phytosterols and phytoestrogens. Soya beans, in particular, are rich in phyto-estrogens. Many pulses, however, contain toxins which are destroyed only by long, slow cooking.*

THE ADVANTAGES OF PLANT-DERIVED FOODS

Vegetarians consistently have lower incidences of cancer, cardiovascular disease and other chronic degenerative diseases. At first this was attributed to a diet containing little saturated fat. Then the benefits of a high-fibre diet were identified, and now it seems that there are multiple factors in plant food that help the body cope with every menace the environment holds, from micro-organisms to harmful chemicals. The best advice seems to be to adopt a diet based primarily on vegetables, fruit and wholegrains. People who are unable or unwilling to eat sufficient fruit and vegetables should consider taking special freeze-dried fruit and vegetable extracts. These supplements are becoming increasingly popular as an easy way of providing the body with 'plant protection'. As well as vitamins and minerals, plants contain the following beneficial substances:

Carotenoids are the fat-soluble yellow, orange and red pigments found in many different fruits and vegetables. There are over 500 different carotenoids (the most well-known ones being betacarotene, alphacarotene, lycopene, lutein and zeaxanthin). Different carotenoids offer different health benefits, amongst them a reduction in the risk of cancers and protection against cataract development and cardiovascular disease. Recent evidence suggests that the different carotenoids have a combined effect far superior to the effects of single, high-dose supplements. In other words, no single supplement, such as betacarotene, can replace the protective effect of the full range of carotenoids. While eating foods rich in carotenoids is advised, supplements containing mixed carotenoids/carotenes are also recommended.

Dietary fibre is vital to the digestive process and the health of the bowel. There are two types: soluble and insoluble. Soluble fibre (found in oats, barley, pulses and fruit) improves bowel transit time, protects against bowel cancer and improves blood sugar and cholesterol profiles. Wheat fibre (bran) is insoluble; although it does not positively affect sugar or cholesterol levels, it is the best treatment for constipation.

Phytosterols/sterols and sterolins. The crucial function of these essential plant fats is immune system modulation. They not only stimulate underactivity (helping in the treatment of cancer, AIDS and chronic infections), but also help control inappropriate immune system activity which can lead to auto-immune disorders (such as rheumatoid arthritis) and allergies (such as hayfever, asthma, eczema and food allergies). They also normalize prostate function. As phytosterols are bound to plant fibre, they are easily lost in refining processes, and many people's diets are deficient. Several herbs (such as Saw palmetto) as well as nuts, seeds and pulses are rich sources. A 20 mg supplement of both sterols and sterolins (such as Moducare, which has been scientifically tested) three times daily is advised to restore and regulate immune function, or 1 tbsp unrefined soya lecithin granules three times daily.

Phytoestrogens are a type of phytosterol present in many plant foods and herbs. They act to balance the effects of oestrogen on the body, making them useful for treating menstrual problems, the menopause and hormone-dependent cancers.

Bioflavonoids (flavonoids/flavonols) are compounds which enhance the activity of vitamin C. They are potent antioxidants, neutralizing all types of free radicals (p. 23). They have a unique ability to protect and regenerate collagen, which is present throughout the body in the connective tissue of skin, cartilage, tendons, ligaments, etcetera. They can cross the blood brain barrier and offer direct protection to the central nervous system, preventing mental deterioration. They strengthen and tone capillary walls, reducing bruising, the severity of sports injuries and the development of varicose veins. Quercetin inhibits the production of histamine and is thus useful in controlling allergic reactions (such as hayfever).

Well-known flavonoids include proanthocyanidins, anthocyanidins and catechins (which are all fifty times more potent than vitamin E and twenty times more potent than vitamin C), as well as rutin, hesperidin, quercetin, curcumin and silymarin.

Recent research has demonstrated that the beneficial effects of many herbs and foods are directly related to their flavonoid content. Bioflavonoids are widely present in fruits and vegetables, especially in the skins, pith and seeds. A mixture of bioflavonoids is recommended – take 250 mg twice daily between meals.

Phytonutrients (phytochemicals). This is a term used to cover the multitude of other substances present in plants which do not fall into any category but have widespread health benefits. These include antiviral, antibacterial and antifungal properties, antioxidant and anti-cancer activity, anti-inflammatory and expectorant effects, immune system stimulation and cholesterol reduction.

THE CHOLESTEROL QUESTION

Despite its bad reputation, cholesterol is vital for health and is a component of most body tissues, including the brain, nervous system, liver and blood. In fact, most cholesterol in the blood is produced by the liver and is not from dietary sources.

There are two main types of cholesterol: HDL (high density lipoprotein) and LDL (low density lipoprotein). The HDL cholesterol is now recognized as beneficial (H for healthy) and high levels confer protection against atherosclerosis (the deposition of cholesterol on the arterial walls). HDL cholesterol acts as a regulator, carrying excess cholesterol back to the liver where it is destroyed and then excreted. Low levels of HDL cholesterol are the most critical indicator of heart disease risk – HDL levels below 15% of the total cholesterol level are considered to be dangerous. LDL cholesterol is the bad type (L for lethal), and the greater the ratio of LDL to HDL the greater the risk of cardiovascular disease.

Below: *Onions, garlic, olive oil, barley and oats have the beneficial effect of lowering the levels of harmful LDL cholesterol in the blood, while raising the levels of the protective HDL cholesterol. Cholesterol-lowering foods can work in two ways: they can prevent the absorption of dietary cholesterol and they can produce substances which switch off liver synthesis of cholesterol. A high intake of saturated fat increases liver synthesis of the unhealthy LDL cholesterol.*

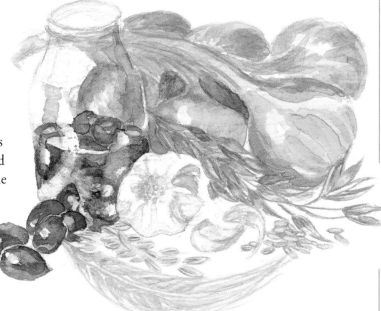

COMMON SYMPTOMS OF FATTY ACID DEFICIENCY

Fatigue

Grogginess on awakening

Depression

Headaches

Dry skin

Dandruff

Dry eyes

Brittle nails

Cold hands and feet

Fluid retention

FACTS ABOUT FATS

All dietary fats are composed of many different fatty acids, which can be either saturated or unsaturated (this includes polyunsaturated and monounsaturated fats). Fats which are solid at room temperature (lard, butter, meat fat, cocoa butter) contain mostly saturated fatty acids, whereas fats which are liquid at room temperature (vegetable oils) contain mostly unsaturated fatty acids.

A high consumption of saturated fats is associated with a wide range of serious health problems. Margarine and vegetable shortening are made by artificially saturating (hydrogenating) vegetable oils. This process involves great heat and leads to the formation of trans fatty acids, which are unhealthy. All artificially saturated fats should be excluded from the diet. Unsaturated fats, depending on the type, quantity and quality, are considered more beneficial.

The metabolism of essential fatty acids

Only two essential fatty acids, both of which are polyunsaturated, need to be supplied in the diet. These are linoleic acid (an omega 6 fatty acid) and alpha-linolenic acid (an omega 3 fatty acid). All the other crucial fatty acids can be made by the body, provided sufficient nutrients are present, especially vitamins B_3, B_6, C, magnesium, zinc and selenium. A high consumption of saturated (including artificially saturated) fats and alcohol interferes with this metabolism of fatty acids. Faulty fatty acid metabolism has been implicated in the development of cancer, heart disease, diabetes, obesity, arthritis, auto-immune disorders, allergies, skin problems, menstrual problems, psychiatric disorders, hyperactivity, gastro-intestinal problems and defective immune response.

IMPORTANT VEGETABLE OILS

OIL	SATURATED	MONOUNSATURATED	POLYUNSATURATED	LA (OMEGA 6)	LNA (OMEGA 3)
Canola (rapeseed)	7.1%	58.9%	29.6%	20.3%	9.3%
Olive	13.5%	73.7%	8.4%	7.9%	0.6%
Flaxseed	4.0%	22.0%	74.0%	17.0%	57.0%
Corn	12.7%	24.2%	58.7%	58.0%	0.7%
Safflower	9.6%	12.6%	73.4%	73.0%	0.2%
Soyabean	14.4%	23.3%	57.9%	51.0%	6.8%

Oils high in monounsaturated fats, such as olive and canola oil, are much more stable than others and are recommended for general use. All oils should be cold-pressed (a type of mechanical extraction that does not involve chemicals or heat) and refrigerated in a dark container. Heat, light, air and refining processes all destroy the essential fatty acids and lead to the production of free radicals (p. 23). The more polyunsaturated the oil, the quicker it spoils. Coconut and palm oils are extremely high in saturated fat and should be avoided. Do not re-use oils which have been heated, as these are high in harmful free radicals and trans fatty acids, and avoid all commercially fried foods.

LA (linoleic acid): omega 6 series

LA (linoleic acid) is widespread in vegetables, wholegrains and vegetable oils. The body can convert LA to GLA (gamma-linolenic acid) and AA (arachidonic acid). (GLA is also found in breastmilk, and in borage, blackcurrant and evening primrose seeds. AA is found in eggs, dairy products and meat.)

GLA is needed to make an important series 1 prostaglandin, which acts to lower blood pressure, thin the blood and inhibit cholesterol production, inflammatory reaction and abnormal cell proliferation. It stimulates the immune system, enhances the effect of insulin and benefits brain function.

GLA can also be converted to AA, which is used to make leukotrienes and a series 2 prostaglandin, both of which are involved in inflammatory processes and the generation of pain. They also make the blood more likely to clot – a vital process if you have injured yourself. However, the production of these leukotrienes and series 2 prostaglandins is increased by a high animal-fat diet (a rich source of AA), upsetting the critical balance between the anti-inflammatory series 1 prostaglandins and the pro-inflammatory series 2 prostaglandins and potentially leading to chronic health problems.

LNA (alpha-linolenic acid): omega 3 series

The richest source of LNA (alpha-linolenic acid) is flaxseed oil. Smaller quantities are found in spinach, walnuts, soya beans, wholegrains and rapeseed (canola) oil.

LNA can be converted to EPA (eicosapentaenoic acid), also present in certain seafoods. EPA is needed to make series 3 prostaglandins and other substances which have beneficial effects similar to the series 1 prostaglandins (see above). Series 3 prostaglandins also appear to be more effective at limiting the production of the pro-inflammatory series 2 prostaglandins and leukotrienes.

Good sources of essential fatty acids

Flaxseed offers one of the healthiest ways to remedy an essential fatty acid deficiency. Take 1 tbsp of cold-pressed oil from organically grown flaxseed daily or 2 tbsp freshly ground flaxseed (unground flaxseed cannot be digested). Flaxseed oil is highly unsaturated and therefore easily oxidized. Keep flaxseed oil in a dark container and store in a refrigerator. Do not use flaxseed oil for cooking. **Note:** Flaxseed is also known as linseed, but the freely available linseed oil used to oil furniture and cricket bats is highly toxic and should never be swallowed.

Borage (starflower), blackcurrant seed and evening primrose oils are rich sources of **GLA**. Borage oil contains 24% GLA and blackcurrant seed oil 18%, while evening primrose oil contains 10%. Supplements are indicated for people who appear unable to convert LA into GLA even if all the conditions are correct. A four- to six-week trial of 500 mg borage/blackcurrant seed oil or 1 000 mg evening primrose oil twice daily will establish whether this is a cause of your problem.

CAUTION

People who suffer from epilepsy should not take any GLA-rich supplements unless under medical supervision.

ESSENTIAL FATTY ACIDS

Most Western diets are skewed in favour of omega 6 fatty acids and are deficient in omega 3 fatty acids. To remedy this, reduce the intake of animal fats and oils rich in omega 6 fatty acids, and increase the intake of foods rich in the omega 3 fatty acids, such as flaxseed and oily fish.

CAUTION

Anyone taking anticoagulant medications should not take EPA-rich supplements, as they thin the blood.

Fish, particularly oily saltwater fish such as mackerel, salmon, tuna, sturgeon, herring, anchovy, sardine and freshwater trout, contains high amounts of the healthy omega 3 fatty acids (but fish commercially raised in ponds are very low in omega 3 fatty acids). One to two servings a week of omega 3-rich fish halve the risk of heart disease.

Fish oil supplements are derived from certain fish and can be a convenient way to boost EPA levels. Fish oil can, however, be a concentrated source of pollutants and free radicals (p. 23), and long-term supplementation may be unsafe. Supplements of 2 g daily are generally recommended. Note that fish liver oil supplements are not the same thing: they are good sources of vitamins A and D, both of which may be harmful in excess, but contain little EPA.

COFFEE AND TEA – HEALTHY OR NOT?

A cup of strong tea contains roughly 50 mg of caffeine, that of coffee 100 mg. (Smaller but still substantial amounts of caffeine are present in chocolate and cola drinks). Pharmacological effects become significant with doses exceeding 200 mg. Caffeine has been implicated as a cause in one or more of the following conditions: anxiety, insomnia, restlessness (including restless leg syndrome), irritability, panic attacks, depression, cardiovascular problems, palpitations, muscle tremors, withdrawal headaches, indigestion, diarrhoea, urinary problems (especially frequent urination), PMS, painful, lumpy breasts and perspiration problems. In addition, caffeine causes a change in brain wave pattern leading to a poorer quality of sleep with fewer periods of deep sleep.

If you suffer from any of these problems it is best to cut ʹout caffeine-containing drinks and foods completely and to drink decaffeinated varieties or herbal tea substitutes (rooibos or chicory). Decaffeinated coffee may still cause indigestion.

However, there are beneficial effects related to caffeine which partly explain the widespread popularity of tea and coffee. Caffeine significantly improves mental performance, mood and physical endurance. (It is, in fact, far superior to many of the drugs banned in sporting events.) It also dilates the bronchial tubes – a beneficial effect for asthmatics. Despite its caffeine content, tea, especially unfermented green tea, has a high flavonoid content and is associated with a whole range of health benefits (p. 107).

Below: *As few as two cups of coffee a day may cause health problems. Caffeine, a stimulant found in coffee, is a vaso-constrictor, which narrows blood vessels thus reducing circulation and raising blood pressure.*

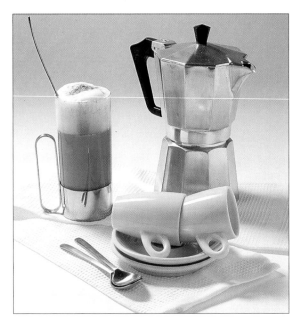

CLINICAL ECOLOGY: THE STUDY OF HOW FOODS AND CHEMICALS IN OUR ENVIRONMENT CAN MAKE US ILL

People are becoming increasingly sensitive to common foods and chemicals in the environment. A diet high in processed and chemically contaminated foods coupled with a high level of environmental pollution is taking its toll on human health.

If you experience any of the following symptoms, which typically wax and wane, you could have a food or chemical sensitivity: asthma, allergic rhinitis (hayfever), urticaria, eczema, sinusitis, recurrent tonsillitis, migraine, abnormal sweating, indigestion, abdominal bloating after a meal, colic, alternating diarrhoea and constipation, fluid retention, weak bladder, muscle and joint pain, obesity, depression, agitation with bounding pulse, panic attacks, irritability, inability to concentrate, behavioural and psychological disturbances, dizziness and fatigue. Alcohol intolerance and food cravings are strong indicators of food allergy.

Asthma, eczema, urticaria and hayfever are disorders associated with the classic allergy response, which is immediate and involves the body producing raised levels of antibodies in response to a normally harmless substance (such as pollen). This stimulates the release of histamine which, in turn, increases skin redness and swelling and constricts the bronchii in the lungs.

Below: *Pesticides and herbicides are used as a matter of course in modern agriculture and contaminate most of our food and water. Not only do they interfere with nutrient absorption and vital biochemical processes, they also generate harmful free radicals (p. 23). Make an effort to obtain organically grown and reared food instead.*

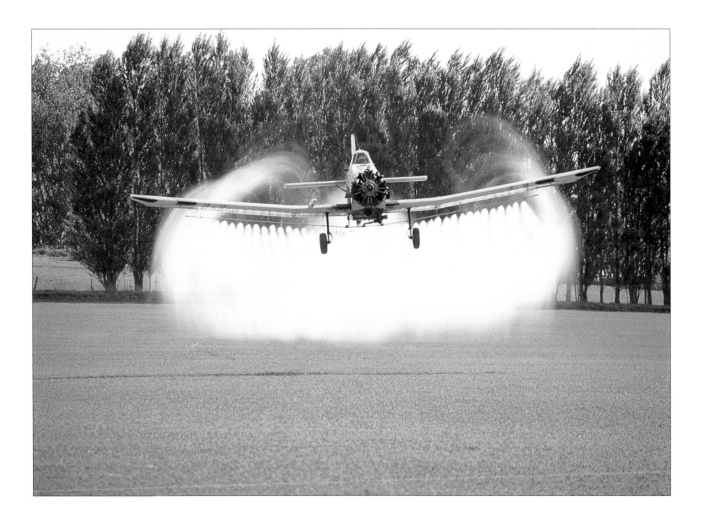

SUPPLEMENTS TO HELP OVERCOME AN ALLERGY

Multivitamin and mineral supplement (p. 31)

Vitamin C 200 mg twice daily

Zinc 15 mg on an empty stomach

Flaxseed oil 1 tbsp

Phytosterol supplement (p. 14) as directed

Acidophilus supplement and golden seal or garlic to control microbial overgrowth

SALT

The average salt intake in a Western diet is estimated to be 10–20 times in excess of the body's requirements. This has directly harmful consequences for up to 20% of the population, who are 'salt-sensitive'. For these people, excess sodium will cause increased fluid retention (putting strain on the heart and kidneys) and increased blood pressure. In addition, the more salt we eat the more potassium we require, so a high salt intake may lead to a potassium deficiency. Salt intake should be reduced by everyone, particularly young children.

ALCOHOL

Alcohol adversely affects almost every vitamin, many minerals and the metabolism of essential fatty acids. People with a high alcohol intake (anything over 2–3 drinks a day, where one drink is equal to a half pint of beer, a glass of wine or a single measure of spirits) are often malnourished. Sustained high alcohol intake is associated with damage to the liver, nervous system, brain and heart. It also increases the incidence of obesity, gout, fetal abnormality and cancer of the liver, breast, oesophagus, larynx or mouth.

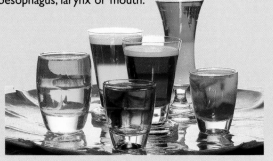

However, many food and chemical allergies do not follow this classic pathway. Reactions may be delayed, intermittent or chronic. It is not yet understood how the allergy develops, but there is evidence that semi-digested food and chemical molecules escape directly into the bloodstream because of increased permeability of the gut (the so-called 'leaky gut syndrome'). Once in the bloodstream they cause an immune response different to the classic allergy response. This can then lead to any of the problems described above.

Food and chemical allergies may develop slowly, but they are more usually precipitated by some form of stress, such as a prolonged viral illness, surgery, a change in the bowel microflora due to antibiotic treatment, incomplete digestion, nutritional deficiencies or emotional stress. An allergy may also be due to an enzyme deficiency (as is the case with lactose intolerance) or an adverse biochemical reaction to a food constituent (as is the case with migraine).

Many of these symptoms may also be due to other more serious causes. Food or chemical allergy should only be suspected if all other causes have been excluded.

Many food or chemical allergies are 'masked', as the person can often feel temporarily better after eating or being exposed to the offending substance – much as an alcoholic will feel temporarily better from alcohol.

Substance 'challenge'

The easiest way to determine an allergy or intolerance is to exclude the suspected substance for a minimum of ten days. During this time the symptoms, which may initially worsen, should clear. An allergy will be confirmed if a 'challenge' with the substance (eating or inhaling it) reproduces the symptoms within a couple of hours (although it may sometimes take a day). If you exclude several substances together, you should challenge with one substance at a time and leave at least two days' interval before challenging with another. The following foods and chemicals are most commonly implicated: dairy products (cow's milk, butter, cream, cheese and yoghurt), gluten (found in wheat, rye, oats and barley), eggs, sugar, corn, coffee, tea, yeast, chocolate, citrus fruit, alcohol, tartrazine, sulphur preservatives, natural gas, tobacco smoke, aerosol chemicals and formaldehyde.

People with serious conditions should consult a clinical ecologist before conducting a substance challenge, as the challenge may produce violent symptoms. Professional advice should be sought regarding suitable substitutes for dairy products if they are being excluded from a baby's diet. Severe exclusion diets should not be continued for longer than 3–4 weeks without obtaining professional advice regarding a balanced diet.

Aside from strict avoidance, a healthy diet, appropriate supplements and a stress management regime may lessen the allergy. Some people find that they can tolerate small amounts of the responsible substance (once every four to seven days) after a period of avoidance. Others discover that they can eat certain allergen foods if they have been organically grown or raised. In this case it is obviously the chemicals in the food, rather than the food itself, that are responsible. Special dilutions made by clinical ecologists of the offending substances can help, especially if it is impossible to avoid the chemical. Homeopathic preparations of the substances have also been found to be helpful.

Many people with food allergies, especially multiple ones, produce insufficient digestive secretions. If gastrointestinal disturbances (bloating, discomfort, flatulence, indigestion, and so on) feature prominently, it is worth taking a course of the following for one month: a digestive enzyme complex and hydrochloric acid supplements, as directed by the manufacturer. If you experience warmth or discomfort, reduce the dosage of hydrochloric acid.

A PROCESS OF ELIMINATION

When you are excluding a particular food, it is important to be aware of hidden sources of that food. For instance, if you are excluding dairy products and using margarine, check that the margarine does not contain whey. If excluding wheat, check the labels of all processed foods carefully and avoid them if starch is mentioned, unless you can check that the source of the starch is from something other than wheat. When dining out, be wary of sauces and soups, many of which have added flour.

COMMON FOOD ALLERGENS

The major food allergies are to those foods we eat most often (usually those eaten every day and at every meal). In order to prevent the development or worsening of food allergies, it is important to try to rotate different foods. This is especially important when weaning a baby and feeding young children. A detailed food diary may help you to pinpoint allergens, especially if you rotate different foods and keep an accurate record of your symptoms.

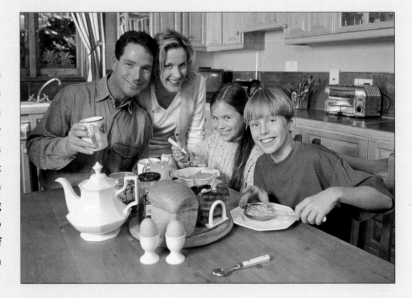

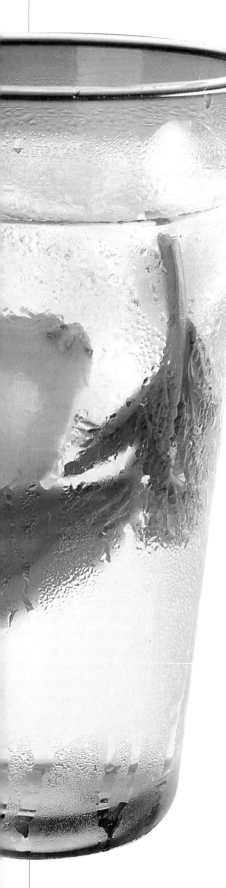

FASTING

Fasting has ancient origins as a therapy. Naturopaths have always recommended fasting for fevers and acute gastrointestinal upsets. Many of us instinctively refrain from solid food when we feel unwell.

Liquids, either spring water, fresh juices or herbal teas, must always be taken regularly during a fast. Short fasts (two days) can safely be carried out by healthy adults without supervision. Pregnant women, children and the elderly should only fast under professional supervision.

Fasting is believed to stimulate the body's innate healing processes. It also provides the liver, the main detoxifying organ of the body, with time to deal with accumulated toxins. Fasting people often experience headaches, diarrhoea and bad breath. These usually disappear by the end of the second day and become less severe if short fasts are undertaken monthly. The fast should always be broken gradually with simple food such as steamed vegetables and salad. Mono fasts, such as eating only grapes, have become popular for treating long-standing chronic degenerative conditions. These should be professionally supervised.

OTHER ANTIOXIDANTS

MELATONIN

Melatonin, a very powerful brain antioxidant, is produced by the pineal gland in the brain and, amongst other functions, regulates sleep. Production is stimulated by darkness; almost constant exposure to bright electric light has reduced melatonin production and is thought to be partly responsible for increased levels of senility and brain malfunction. Supplements are effective in relieving insomnia and jet lag (p. 136). It is recommended that dosage is limited to 1 g or less daily, and that they are taken 2–3 hours before you wish to fall asleep. Note that in some countries, supplements are available on prescription only.

CO-ENZYME Q10

This is an antioxidant substance widely present in foodstuffs (soya, wholegrains, fish, nuts, etc.). It can be manufactured by the body if adequate vitamin E is present. Supplements have been found to improve heart function, diabetes, AIDS and Alzheimer's disease and reduce high blood pressure. Emulsified forms of co-enzyme Q10 are best, and a daily dosage of 30–90 mg is recommended.

Left: *Regular consumption of water is essential to life. Sadly, over 800 different water contaminants have been identified, ranging from pesticides and hormones to toxic metals such as lead, cadmium and aluminium. Bottled or filtered water is advised (reverse osmosis purification systems or activated carbon filters are recommended).*

FREE RADICALS, OXIDATIVE STRESS AND THE ROLE OF ANTIOXIDANTS

Oxygen is essential for life, but our dependence on it comes at a price. By-products of our normal metabolism include a group of highly unstable molecules of oxygen referred to as free radicals (peroxide, hydroxyl and superoxide radicals) and singlet oxygen. These 'reactive oxygen species' rapidly react with (oxidize) and damage substances throughout the body (such as proteins, fats and DNA) to form new, unstable molecules which can also be referred to as free radicals. These react with further molecules, causing a chain reaction of free radical formation and leaving behind a path of altered and damaged molecules.

This destructive process would go on indefinitely until the body was irreparably harmed if nature had not provided a defence against free radical oxidation. Certain enzymes produced by the body (glutathione peroxidase and superoxide dismutase) deactivate free radicals. However, the production of these enzymes is dependent on adequate supplies of zinc, copper, manganese and selenium in the diet. In addition, vitamins A, C and E, zinc, selenium, various carotenoids, bioflavonoids and co-enzyme Q10, all of which are widely present in foodstuffs, are effective antioxidants which neutralize free radicals. In the process these nutrients are inactivated and eliminated from the body. They therefore need to be continually supplied by the diet. As some antioxidants neutralize only one type of free radical, the full range needs to be present to offer complete protection.

If the body is unable to match the production of free radicals with anti-oxidants it is said to be in a state of oxidative stress. Free radicals then run amok, damaging cells and leading to inflammation, impaired immunity, infection and eventually cancer, cardiovascular disease, cataracts, arthritis and a range of degenerative diseases and conditions associated with the ageing process. Stress, infections, drugs, anaesthesia, cigarette smoke, environmental pollution, poor nutrition, the presence of too much iron and copper and radiation (including from UV light, X-rays and so on) all contribute to the production of free radicals. This extra load, combined with widespread nutritional deficiencies, means that many of us are in a state of oxidative stress and are ageing and degenerating faster than we should. Statistics of chronic disease certainly confirm this trend, which can be easily reversed by simple dietary changes and the use of supplements.

AMINO ACIDS

Single high doses of amino acids are not recommended generally. However, nutritional deficiencies and metabolic errors can lead to deficiencies in one or more of the synthesized amino acids. Glutathione and its pre-cursor N-acetyl cysteine appear to be two of the most important, as both protect against oxidative damage within the cells and combine with chemical toxins so that they can be excreted. Supplements of either have been found useful for people with chemical allergies, alcohol poisoning (hangover), chronic fatigue, AIDS and after chemotherapy. The recommended dosage is 500 mg twice daily.

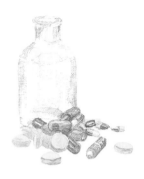

VITALITY FROM VITAMINS AND MINERALS

Once scientists had identified the vitamins and minerals that are essential to health, they set about working out the minimum amount of each required by the body on a daily basis to prevent the development of deficiency syndromes such as scurvy (vitamin C deficiency) and beriberi (vitamin B_1 deficiency). Different terms are used to refer to these amounts, including recommended daily allowance (RDA) or reference nutrient intake (RNI), and they soon gained wide acceptance as a guarantee of good health. The allowances are now being challenged on three counts.

Firstly, whereas gross deficiency is now quite rare in developed countries, evidence is mounting that marginal deficiencies are pervasive and widespread. During the sub-clinical (marginal) deficiency stage, essential biochemical reactions are impaired owing to inadequate cellular levels of vitamins and minerals. This affects the body in numerous ways without necessarily leading to recognizable physical signs of deficiency. Brain function is often the first to be compromised, especially by a lack of B and C vitamins. Fatigue, depression, anxiety and insomnia are some of the many proven symptoms of marginal deficiency syndromes. Marginal nutritional status also adversely affects the body's immune system, and its ability to recover from surgery and disease and to metabolize drugs and environmental toxins.

Secondly, while allowance is made for the fact that adolescents and pregnant and lactating women need more vitamins and minerals, the huge variation in individual needs is not taken into account. Some people have significantly higher requirements because they cannot absorb and utilize vitamins and minerals as well as others can. During periods of physiological stress (from surgical operations, infections, drug and

Above: *When you are in good health you should feel vital and energetic. If you cannot remember when you last felt like this you may well be deficient in a number of vitamins and minerals. Appropriate supplements, coupled with a healthy diet and lifestyle, will help to restore vitality.*

hormone treatment, high alcohol intake, smoking and chemically contaminated food and air) and psychological stress (such as anxiety, worry or grief), daily requirements increase dramatically.

Thirdly, extensive research into the biochemical involvement of vitamins and various minerals throughout the body has made it clear that, apart from merely keeping deficiency disorders at bay, vitamins and minerals play an active part in preventing disease and health disorders, **but only if they are taken in amounts far exceeding the recommended daily allowances.** For example, vitamin E can help prevent heart attacks but never at RDA levels, and vitamin B_6 relieves premenstrual tension, but only in doses at least twenty five times greater than the RDA.

TOXIC METALS

Chronic low-level exposure to a range of metals such as lead, cadmium, aluminium and mercury has been linked to a range of health disorders. Lead toxicity is a causative factor in stillbirths, developmental abnormalities, nervous system problems, immune dysfunction, cancer, heart disease, high blood pressure, learning and behavioural disorders as well as many non-specific symptoms of ill-health. Cadmium, present in cigarettes and many processed foods, wreaks havoc throughout the body by displacing zinc, a commonly deficient mineral, from crucial enzyme systems. Aluminium, used in cooking pots, cans, packaging materials and added to certain deodorants, flour, salt and antacid preparations, accumulates in the body and exerts its toxic effect primarily on the central nervous system. It has been implicated in the development of Alzheimer's disease and other forms of dementia. Mercury is also toxic to the central nervous system, producing a range of mental and neurological problems. (Mercury vapour has been measured in the mouths of people with amalgam fillings and many people have reported relief from chronic symptoms after their removal.)

Vitamins C, D and E, calcium, magnesium, zinc, iron, chromium and selenium reduce the absorption and encourage the excretion of toxic metals and chemicals.

A seaweed/algae supplement (fucus/laminaria species) is recommended, in powder or tablet form, to be taken as directed by the manufacturer and with meals. Alginate is a complex carbohydrate component of the cell walls of seaweed and cannot be broken down by the human digestive system. It has a unique ability to bind with harmful metals (such as lead, mercury, cadmium, radium and strontium), which are then excreted. It also prevents the reabsorption of any toxic metals which have been stored by the body and then released into the intestines.

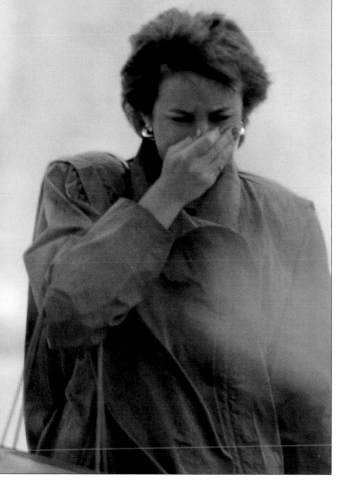

VITAMIN/ MINERAL	RNI/RDA RANGE	THERAPEUTIC DOSAGE RANGE	HEALTHY FOOD SOURCES
VITAMIN A: antioxidant; fat-soluble CAUTION: Toxic above 25 000 IU	2 300–3 300 IU	5 000–10 000 IU during pregnancy: 5 000–8 000 IU	dairy products; liver
BETACAROTENE: antioxidant; water-soluble; non-toxic; converted to vitamin A as required by the body	not established	not established, but up to 15 mg (equivalent to 25 000 IU)	orange and red fruit and vegetables (apricots, mangoes, paw paws, peaches, melons, tomatoes, corn, carrots, sweet potatoes, squash); green leafy vegetables
VITAMIN B COMPLEX: water-soluble; generally non-toxic CAUTION: Vitamin B_6 intake should not exceed 300 mg Vitamin B-related substances	B_1/thiamin: 1–1.5 mg B_2/riboflavin: 1.3–1.7 mg B_3/niacin/nicotinic acid/ nicotinamide: 17–19 mg B_5/pantothenic acid/calcium D pantothenate: 4–7 mg B_6/pyridoxine: 1.4–2 mg folic acid: 200 mcg B_{12}: 1.5–2 mcg biotin: 100–200 mcg choline: not established inositol: not established	B_1/thiamin: 10–50 mg B_2/riboflavin: 10–50 mg B_3/niacin/nicotinic acid/ nicotinamide: 50–150 mg B_5/pantothenic acid/calcium D pantothenate: 40–100 mg B_6/pyridoxine: 15–50 mg folic acid: 500–1 000 mcg B_{12}: 10–50 mcg biotin: 150–300 mcg choline: 2–100 mg inositol: 30–100 mg	wholegrains (brown rice, wheat, millet); pulses (soya beans, lentils); mackerel; herring NOTE: Vitamin B_{12} occurs in animal food sources only True vitamin B_{12} is not present in algae
VITAMIN C: antioxidant; water-soluble CAUTION: New research suggests doses well above 500 mg daily may harm basic aspects of cellular biochemistry	40–60 mg	100 mg–500 mg	most fruit and vegetables (berries, citrus, guavas, green and red peppers, broccoli, brussels sprouts and kale); rosehips and acerola cherries are richest known natural sources
VITAMIN D: fat-soluble CAUTION: Toxic if more than 25 000 IU are taken daily	up to 200 IU	100–400 IU	made by the body when exposed to sunlight; fatty fish; eggs; dairy products
VITAMIN E: antioxidant; fat-soluble CAUTION: Avoid high-dose supplements if taking anticoagulants. Daily supplements above 600 IU are not recommended	7.5 IU	100–600 IU	nuts (almonds, brazils, hazels); seeds; pulses; wholegrains
CALCIUM Calcium absorption is improved by the presence of vitamin D and magnesium, but impaired by a high fat and protein diet CAUTION: Dolomite and bonemeal are not recommended	700–800 mg	200–1 500 mg	pulses (soya); nuts; seeds (sesame); green leafy vegetables; kelp/ seaweed; apple juice; molasses; dairy products (however, these may cause food allergies and lactose intolerance)

GOOD SUPPLEMENT FORMS	DEFICIENCY SYMPTOMS	FURTHER TREATMENT INDICATIONS
dried liver; fish liver oils (p. 18, caution)	frequent colds and infections; poor night vision; dry eyes; rough, dry, scaly and blemished skin; fatigue	bronchitis; asthma; measles; diarrhoea; brittle nails; mouth ulcers, pimples and spots
freeze-dried fruit and vegetable extracts; mixed carotenoid supplement (including betacarotene)	as above	as above, and cancer; heart disease; cataracts
slow-release B complex formulation; nutritional yeast; brewer's yeast; molasses; wheatgerm; lecithin (rich in choline and inositol)	fatigue; irritability; depression; anxiety; panic attacks; personality changes; impaired concentration and memory; chronic headaches; burning, sensitive, gritty eyes; red, greasy skin with scaly, dry patches (combination skin); cracks at corners of mouth; swollen, fissured, shiny tongue; numbness and tingling; burning feet; tender calf muscles; anaemia	stressful situations and jobs; smoking; drinking alcohol; hyperactivity; schizophrenia; infection; post-operative pain; nausea; acne; seborrhoeic dermatitis; gastrointestinal problems; allergies; insomnia; PMS; migraine; asthma; cardiovascular disease
magnesium or calcium ascorbate; ascorbic acid (take chewable forms with meals to avoid erosion of dental enamel)	depression; hysteria; red pimples; bleeding, swollen gums; easy bruising; nosebleeds; slow wound healing; frequent infections	infants whose milk formulas are not supplemented with fruit or vegetables; all infections; cardiovascular disease; cancer; diabetes; arthritis; burns; drug addiction; smoking; allergies; toxic overload
cod liver oil (p. 18, caution)	poor bone and tooth formation; tooth decay; joint pain and stiffness; muscle weakness; bowed legs or waddling gait	vegans; people insufficiently exposed to sunlight (institutionalized people, the elderly, and dark-skinned people living in high latitudes); osteoporosis; arthritis
wheatgerm; choose supplements containing mixed natural tocopherols	associated with impaired immune function and miscarriage	cardiovascular disease; cancer; Alzheimer's disease; infections; burns; scar tissue; irregular menstruation; fibrocystic breast disease; PMS; age spots; infertility
chelated calcium/calcium citrate in effervescent or chewable forms	increased susceptibility to food allergies; asthma; eczema; hayfever; depression; anxiety; panic attacks; nervous tics and twitches; hyperactivity; insomnia	arthritis; cataracts; osteoporosis NOTE: Deficiency increases the body's absorption of toxic metals lead and aluminium (p. 25)

VITAMIN/ MINERALS	RNI/RDI RANGE	THERAPEUTIC DOSAGE RANGE	HEALTHY FOOD SOURCES
POTASSIUM	2 000–5 000 mg	not recommended	salt substitutes containing potassium chloride; fruits (peaches, prunes, raisins, bananas); vegetables (tomatoes); pulses (lima, pinto, soya, chickpeas)
MAGNESIUM Magnesium is commonly deficient in a diet high in refined and processed foods	300–350 mg	200–1 000 mg	green leafy vegetables; wholegrains (wheat, millet); nuts (brazil, cashew, almonds); seeds (sesame); pulses (soya); seafood; molasses; kelp/seaweed

TRACE ELEMENTS

VITAMIN/ MINERALS	RNI/RDI RANGE	THERAPEUTIC DOSAGE RANGE	HEALTHY FOOD SOURCES
IRON Iron absorption is enhanced by vitamin C (100 mg vitamin C with meals can lead to a tenfold increase in the absorption of iron), but inhibited (by up to 80%) by tea or coffee, which should not be taken with meals, especially by those at risk of iron deficiency	8.7–10 mg	not recommended	pulses (peas, beans, lentils); green leafy vegetables (parsley, spinach); wholegrains (rice, wheat, millet); dried fruits (apricots, prunes, raisins); shellfish; egg yolk; organ meats
ZINC: antioxidant CAUTION: Do not exceed 100 mg daily	9.5–15 mg	15–40 mg	wholegrains (brown rice, wheat); pulses (soya); nuts (brazil, cashew); seeds (sunflower, pumpkin); seafood (oysters, crab)
SELENIUM: antioxidant CAUTION: Always to be taken in conjunction with vitamin E	70–75 mcg	50–300 mcg	wholegrains; nuts; seeds; seafood (lobster, oysters, shrimp and cod)
IODINE CAUTION: Excessive levels may aggravate pimples and spots and suppress thyroid function	140–150 mcg	25–100 mcg	wholegrains; seafood (fish and shellfish)
CHROMIUM	25–50 mcg	50–200 mcg	wholegrains; black pepper

NOTE: Other important trace elements, which should be included in a multivitamin and mineral supplement, are copper, manganese, boron and molybdenum. While much is unknown about the function of these and other trace elements (such as vanadium or silicon), they are all required in minute quantities but may be harmful in larger amounts.

GOOD SUPPLEMENT FORMS	DEFICIENCY SYMPTOMS	FURTHER TREATMENT INDICATIONS
none (oral supplements are associated with gastrointestinal problems)	muscular weakness and cramp; irregular heart beat; depression; apathy; fatigue; poor appetite; constipation	high blood pressure; chronic diarrhoea
chelated magnesium; magnesium citrate; magnesium aspartate; magnesium orotate; magnesium oxide	fatigue; anxiety; depression; confusion and disorientation; learning disability; impaired memory; vertigo; hyperactivity; insomnia; muscle cramps; numbness and tingling; tremors; hypoglycaemia; constipation; heart rhythm problems	osteoporosis; joint aches and pains; a range of psychiatric problems; hypertension; kidney stones; PMS; diabetes
increase intake of iron-rich food (see left) and take 100 mg vitamin C with meals to enhance absorption	high-risk groups: pregnant women, women with heavy periods and children and adolescents; anaemia (listlessness, fatigue, palpitations, sore tongue, cracks at corner of mouth, difficulty swallowing, concave nails); poor appetite, growth and mental performance; frequent infections	behavioural disorders in children; food allergy NOTE: Blood tests should confirm deficiency before you begin taking additional iron supplements; self-medication is not recommended as excess iron stimulates free radical formation (p. 23)
nutritional yeast; brewer's yeast; wheatgerm; chelated zinc; zinc orotate; zinc citrate	NOTE: zinc is commonly deficient. infertility; low sperm count; slow growth and delayed sexual maturity; hair loss; dandruff; white spots on nails; frequent infections; slow wound healing; behavioural and psychiatric problems; skin problems; impaired sense of taste, smell and vision; stretchmarks	pimples, spots; psoriasis; burns; skin ulcers; sleep disorders, especially in babies; rheumatoid arthritis; anorexia nervosa; bulimia; alcoholism
nutritional yeast; brewer's yeast; seaweed/kelp; chelated selenium; sodium selenium	deficiency may be associated with liver disease; cancer; heart disease and arthritis	any degenerative condition; food allergy; chemical allergy; infertility; if you live in an area with selenium-deficient soil such as New Zealand or the UK
seaweed/kelp	underactive thyroid gland, characterized by weakness, fatigue, weight gain, dry skin, menorrhagia and constipation	multiple sclerosis; Parkinson's disease; Alzheimer's disease; motor neuron disease
wheatgerm; nutritional yeast; brewer's yeast; GTF chromium	poor blood sugar control; depressed sperm formation	cardiovascular disease; diabetes (type II); hypoglycaemia; obesity

COMMON DEFICIENCIES

The most common deficiencies worldwide, even amongst 'well-nourished' populations, include vitamins A, B_1, B_2, B_6, folic acid, B_{12}, C and E, calcium, magnesium, iron, selenium and zinc. Much of the problem in the West is due to modern food processing methods, long storage and distribution times and farming practices which lead to mineral-depleted soils.

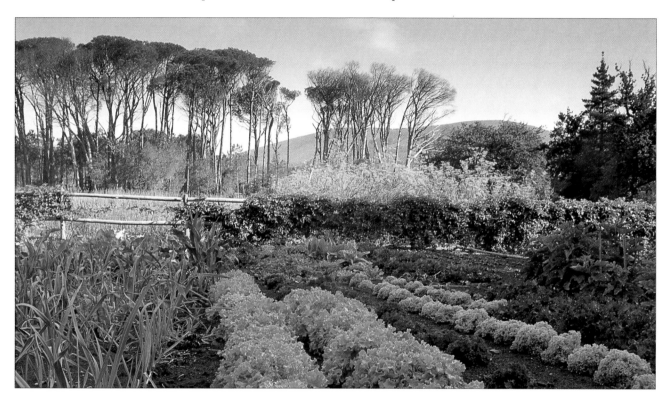

CHELATED MINERALS

Mineral salts are, in general, poorly absorbed by the digestive system. Chelated minerals are those which are bound to an organic molecule such as an amino acid, making them easier to absorb. Most minerals in plant and animal matter occur in chelated form.

TAKING SUPPLEMENTS

General supplements are best taken with meals. Tea, coffee and bran adversely affect mineral absorption and should not be taken at the same time as any supplement. Consult a doctor before giving supplements to any child under two years of age.

Above: *Organically grown produce is much richer in nutrients, particularly the trace elements such as zinc, iron, selenium and manganese, than artificially fertilized food. It is also free of the pesticides which widely contaminate foods of both plant and animal origin. Careful scrubbing or peeling of non-organically grown fruits and vegetables is recommended to remove most surface pesticide residues. However, as many of the pesticides used today are absorbed by the growing plant, they cannot be removed in this manner. These foods can be harmful if they are marketed and eaten before the poison has broken down (during the unsafe period). If you cannot obtain organically grown produce, do not be deterred from eating lots of fruit and vegetables, however, as they come packed full of protective factors which help to neutralize pesticides and other environmental poisons.*

DAILY MULTIVITAMIN AND MINERAL SUPPLEMENT

VITAMIN/MINERAL	CHILD	ADULT
A	1 000–2 000 IU	2 000–5 000 IU
BETACAROTENE	2 mg	2–5 mg
B_1	2–5 mg	5–10 mg
B_2	2–5 mg	5–10 mg
B_3/NIACIN/NICOTINAMIDE	10–25 mg	25–50 mg
B_5/CALCIUM PANTOTHENATE/PANTOTHENIC ACID	5–10 mg	10–20 mg
B_6	2–5 mg	5–10 mg
B_{12}	2–5 mcg	5–10 mcg
FOLIC ACID	100–200 mcg	200–400 mcg
BIOTIN	25–50 mcg	50–100 mcg
CHOLINE	10 mg	25 mg
INOSITOL	10 mg	25 mg
C	50–100 mg	100–150 mg
D	100–200 IU	100–200 IU
E	10–15 IU	15–30 IU
CALCIUM	50–100 mg	50–100 mg
MAGNESIUM	25–50 mg	50–75 mg
ZINC	3–5 mg	5–10 mg
MANGANESE	1–2 mg	2–4 mg
IRON	1–2 mg	3–5 mg
BORON	1 mg	2 mg
COPPER	200–300 mcg	500–1 000 mcg
SELENIUM	25 mcg	50–100 mcg
CHROMIUM	15–20 mcg	20–50 mcg
IODINE	10–25 mcg	20–40 mcg
MOLYBDENUM	10–20 mcg	20–50 mcg

NOTES

- Values given for minerals are elemental.
- The values given here are not absolute but have been selected according to the available evidence.
- IU stands for international unit.
- Calcium and magnesium are often included in multivitamin and mineral supplements but, because of constraints on supplement size, usually not in significant amounts; they should thus be taken together as an additional supplement (magnesium 100–200 mg; calcium 200–400 mg).
- Iron in excess can promote free radical formation (p. 23).
- Where a higher dose of a single B vitamin is indicated, it should always be taken together with a multivitamin and mineral supplement. Additional B complex supplements must include the following: B_1, B_2, B_3, B_5, B_6, B_{12}, folic acid and biotin.
- Extra supplements of zinc are best taken on an empty stomach.
- As so many nutrients are interrelated in function and effect, it is important to use a balanced nutritional supplement.
- Supplements should be free from artificial colorants, flavourants, preservatives and any foods to which you may have an allergy (such as gluten, lactose, yeast or sugar).
- Bioflavonoids and fatty acids GLA/EPA may be included in a general supplement.

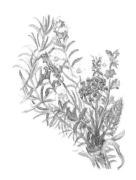

HERBAL HEALING

The use of herbs in the treatment of disease is probably the oldest form of medicine known to man: by 3 000 BC the ancient Egyptians and Chinese already had a sophisticated knowledge of different herbs and their properties. Every culture throughout history has used herbs in one form or another to promote health and treat disease. It has been estimated that even today 75% of the world's population relies on herbalism as the mainstay of treatment.

In the West the use of herbs declined with the advent of the pharmaceutical industry. Initially, the so-called active ingredient was extracted from the herb, for example digitalis from the foxglove and morphine from the 'opium' poppy. The active plant ingredients were then synthesized in a laboratory. Many were added to and changed. Scientists, doctors and pharmaceutical companies believed these chemicals to be superior in every way to the original herb and actively campaigned to have the practice of herbalism banned. One of their main objections to herbal remedies, still a valid criticism today, is that herbs can vary substantially in strength and quality. However, the most important aspect of herbalism – that each herb contains many pharmacologically active ingredients – was overlooked in the zealous pursuit of a single drug to counteract every symptom of a disease.

The presence of a variety of ingredients in each herb has been shown to enhance and broaden the effect: combined, the different active ingredients work together to make the herb far more effective than the synthesized chemical can ever be.

As orthodox medicine battles to cope with the tidal wave of chronic disease and the problem of bacterial resistance to antibiotics, attention has been re-directed to this timeless method of healing.

CAUTION

It is often said that herbal remedies are totally safe. This is untrue. One only has to think of plants like arnica, deadly nightshade *(Atropa belladonna)* and monkshood *(Aconitum napellus)*, which are safe in homeopathic doses, but can be toxic in normal herbal doses. All the herbs recommended in the *Ailment and Treatment Glossary* (from p. 89) are safe for home use, provided you observe the stated dosage and cautionary instructions. If you are gathering your own, be sure to identify the herb correctly. Never gather from the roadside, as herbs will be contaminated with lead and other toxic substances. Obtain all other herbal material from reputable retailers.

COMMERCIALLY AVAILABLE HERBAL PREPARATIONS

Type	Dosage
TINCTURE This is a concentrated extract using alcohol.	Take as directed by the manufacturer.
FREEZE-DRIED/SOLID EXTRACT This is the most concentrated type of herbal extract (as all the liquid solvent is evaporated), and is available in capsule or tablet form. It is highly recommended, as it is cost effective, has long-term chemical stability and is easy to take.	Follow the manufacturer's dosage directions carefully.
STANDARDIZED EXTRACT Although tinctures, fluid extracts and solid extracts are all concentrated, if the herbal source is inferior they may not contain a sufficient quantity of the active ingredients to bring about a physiological effect. Standardized extracts overcome this problem by ensuring that the main active ingredient of each herb is present in a sufficient quantity to achieve a clinical effect. (They are not altered in any other way and still contain the full range of co-factors which enhance and broaden the crucial ingredient's function.) This has made standardized preparations more reliable and increasingly popular. If available, standardized extracts should be used in preference to other forms of a herb in order to guarantee the desired clinical effect.	Take as directed by the manufacturer.

Below: *For a compress,* soak a clean cloth in a bowl of liquid herbal extract (infusion, decoction or diluted tincture 1:20) and apply to affected area.

Below: *Make a poultice* by wrapping in gauze the solid herbal matter retained after you have made an infusion or decoction. Apply to affected area. Use a hot water bottle to maintain the heat.

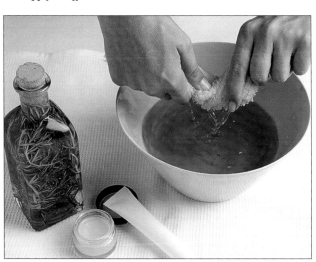

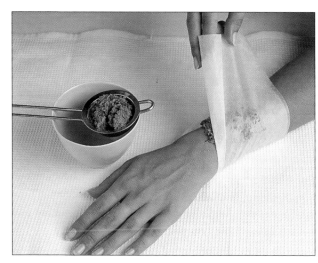

HERBAL PREPARATIONS YOU CAN MAKE AT HOME

Type	Method	Dosage
INFUSION/TEA This method of extraction is suitable for leaves and flowers. **TASTE** If necessary, heat each dose and sweeten with honey (p. 90, caution) or sugar.	Add 500 ml (2 cups) just-boiled water to a total of 30 g (1 oz) dried or 60 g (2 oz) fresh herbs. For a smaller dose, pour 250 ml (1 cup) just-boiled water over 10 ml (2 tsp) dried herbs or 20 ml (4 tsp) fresh herbs. Cover and steep for ten minutes, then strain the infusion. Cover and refrigerate. Make a fresh infusion daily.	ACUTE CONDITIONS **Adults** One wine-glass dose every 30 minutes until relief is obtained **Children under 12 years** Half adult dosage **Infants under 2 years** Quarter adult dosage CHRONIC CONDITIONS **Adults** One wine-glass dose three times daily between meals for at least four weeks **Children under 12 years** Half adult dosage **Infants under two years** Quarter adult dosage
DECOCTION This method of extraction is suitable for bark, berries and roots.	Bring 750 ml (3 cups) cold water and a total of 30 g (1 oz) dried or 60 g (2 oz) fresh herbs to the boil in a non-aluminium pan. Simmer uncovered for 20–30 minutes. Strain, cover and refrigerate.	As for infusion/tea (above)
TINCTURE This method of extraction is suitable for all parts of the plant. As a tincture contains alcohol, which acts as a preservative, it will keep for up to two years. **COMMERCIAL TINCTURES** If taking commercially prepared tinctures, carefully observe the manufacturers' dosage directions, as some makes may vary in strength. For topical applications dilute tincture 1:20 with water.	Place 100 g (4 oz) dried herbs or 200 g (8 oz) fresh herbs in a glass container. Add 500 ml (2 cups) vodka or cane spirit. Cover the container and leave in a cool, dark place for two weeks, shaking occasionally. Strain and decant into clearly labelled dark glass bottles for storage. **Note** To remove alcohol, add tincture drops to hot water, mix and leave to cool before drinking. It is appropriate to apply this practice during pregnancy.	ACUTE CONDITIONS **Adults** 25 drops on the tongue or in a little water every 30 minutes until relief is obtained **Children under 12 years** As above but take 12 drops only **Infants under 2 years** As above but take 2 drops only CHRONIC CONDITIONS **Adults** 25 drops in a little warm water three times daily for at least four weeks **Children under 12 years** As above but take 12 drops only **Infants under 2 years** As above but take 3 drops only

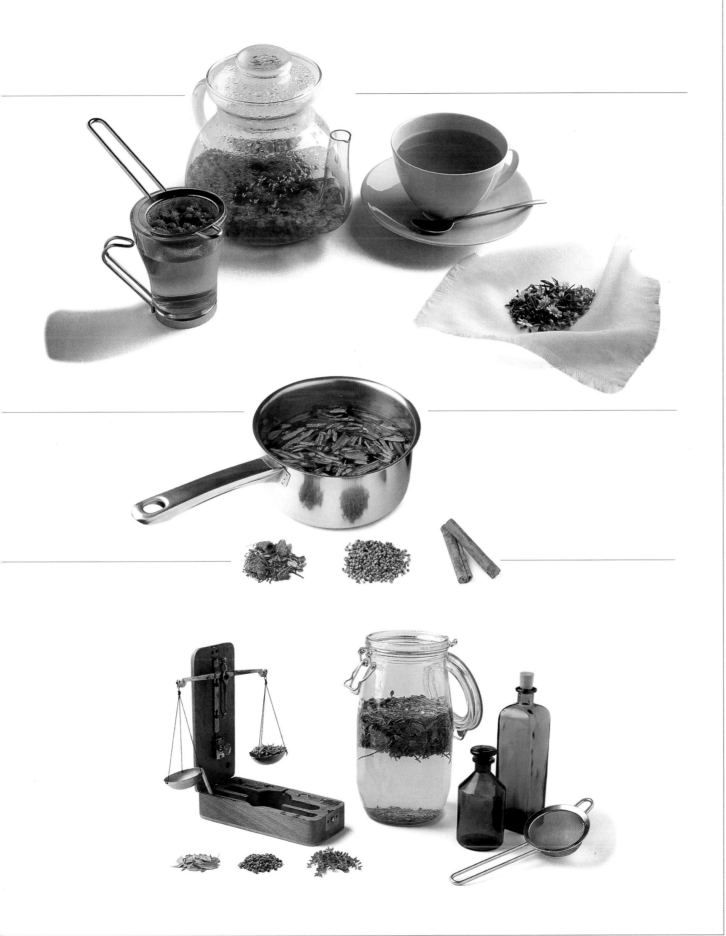

HEALING HERBS FOR THE HOME PHARMACY

Agothosma betulina BUCHU
Part used: leaf
Properties: antimicrobial; diuretic; antispasmodic; sedative
Use for: cystitis; urethritis; gout; colic
Recommended forms: tincture; freeze-dried extract

Allium sativum GARLIC
Part used: bulb
Properties: antioxidant; antimicrobial; expectorant; immune stimulant; decongestant; antimutagenic; anticoagulant; lowers blood pressure and cholesterol levels;
Use for: all infections; cardiovascular disease; high blood pressure
Recommended forms: For all infections add a freshly chopped raw clove to food three times daily or take kyolic garlic capsules. For cardiovascular disease and high blood pressure use fresh or cooked garlic, or 500 mg garlic capsules twice daily.

Aloe vera ALOE VERA
Part used: leaf
Properties: healing; soothing
Use for: sunburn; thermal burns; cuts; sores; inflamed skin; eczema; gastrointestinal inflammation/ulceration
Recommended forms: For skin problems use clear sap or gel direct from leaf, or 90% pure commercial preparation; for gastrointestinal treatment take 1 tsp pure aloe vera juice after meals (use less if dose is laxative).

CAUTION Avoid internal use in pregnancy.

Angelica sinensis DONG QUAI/ CHINESE ANGELICA
Part used: root
Properties: oestrogen balancing; vitamin-rich; female aphrodisiac; immune-stimulant; antimicrobial; anti-bacterial; anti-allergic
Use for: menstrual disorders; menopause; after childbirth as a restorative; general fatigue; anaemia;
Recommended forms: standardized extract; freeze-dried extract

CAUTION Avoid in pregnancy.

Apium graviolens CELERY
Part used: seed
Properties: diuretic; anti-inflammatory
Use for: gout; rheumatoid arthritis; high blood pressure
Recommended forms: decoction; tablets

CAUTION Avoid high doses in pregnancy.
Use only seed sold for medicinal purposes.

Arctostaphylos uva-ursi UVA URSI/BEARBERRY
Part used: leaf
Properties: astringent; antimicrobial
Use for: cystitis; urethritis; prostatitis; heavy menstruation
Recommended forms: tincture; freeze-dried extract

CAUTION Avoid in pregnancy.
Avoid long-term usage.

Arnica montana ARNICA
Part used: flower
Properties: reduces pain, swelling and bruising
Use for: bruises; sprains; sore muscles; sore joints
Recommended forms: cream; ointment; oil; tincture

CAUTION Do not use internally (except in homeopathic remedies).
Do not use on broken skin.

Aspalathus linearis ROOIBOS/REDBUSH
Part used: leaves
Properties: antioxidant; sedative; antispasmodic; anti-inflammatory; anti-allergic
Use for: nervous tension; insomnia; colic; hayfever; asthma; eczema; acne
Recommended form: infusion

Astragalus membranaceous ASTRAGALUS/ HUANG QI
Part used: root
Properties: immune-stimulant; antimutagenic
Use for: run-down people, especially youngsters, who suffer repeated infections
Recommended forms: tincture; freeze-dried extract

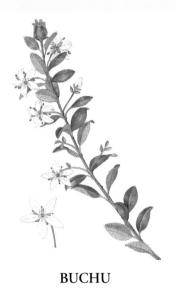

BUCHU

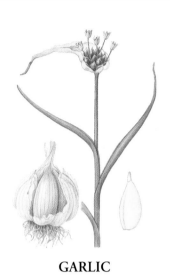

GARLIC

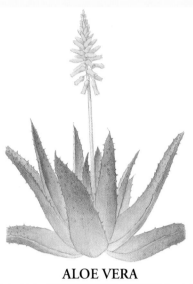

ALOE VERA

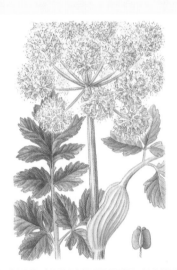

DONG QUAI/CHINESE ANGELICA

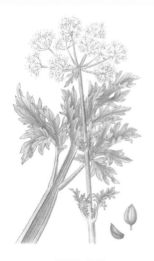

CELERY

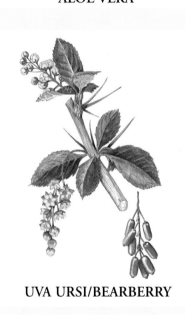

UVA URSI/BEARBERRY

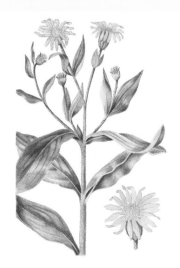

ARNICA

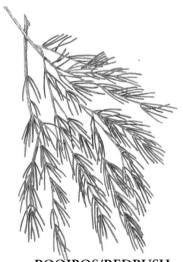

ROOIBOS/REDBUSH

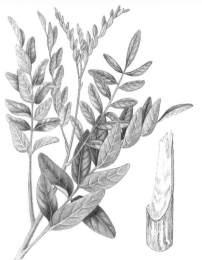

ASTRAGALUS/HUANG QI

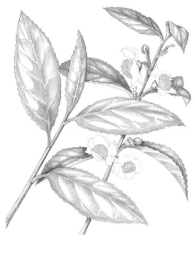

CALENDULA/POT MARIGOLD

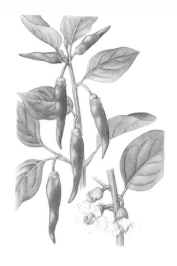
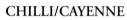

GREEN AND BLACK TEA

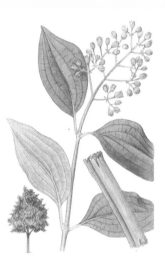

CHILLI/CAYENNE

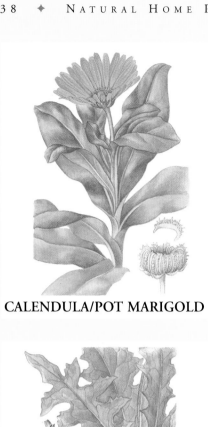

CHICORY

BLACK COHOSH

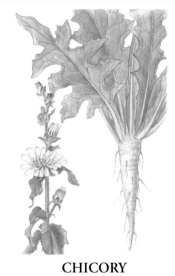

CINNAMON

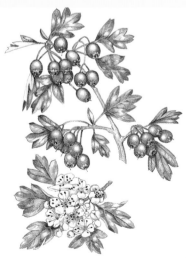

HAWTHORN

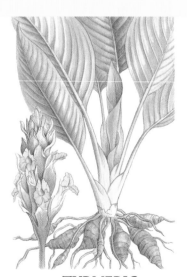

TURMERIC

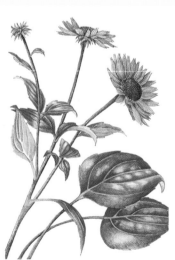

ECHINACEA

Calendula officinalis CALENDULA/ POT MARIGOLD

Part used: flower
Properties: healing; antimicrobial; oestrogen balancing
Use for: cuts; grazes; infected sores; fungal infections; inflammatory skin conditions; dry skin; menstrual problems
Recommended forms: cream; ointment; infusion; tincture

Camellia sinensis GREEN AND BLACK TEA

Part used: leaf
Properties: powerful antioxidant; antimutagenic; lowers blood pressure and cholesterol levels; anticoagulant; strengthens capillaries; antibacterial; antiviral
Use for: cardiovascular disease; high blood pressure; tooth decay; all infections; skin cancer; cancer; AIDS
Recommended form: Infusion (without milk). Green tea is more medicinal than the common fermented black tea. Use decaffeinated varieties.

Capsicum frutescens CHILLI/CAYENNE

Part used: fruit
Properties: expectorant; decongestant; analgesic; anti-inflammatory; anticoagulant; lowers cholesterol; vasodilator
Use for: headache; chronic bronchitis; emphysema; asthma; colds; sinusitis; cardiovascular disease; ulcerative colitis; poor circulation; neuralgia; post-shingles pain; painful muscles; painful joints; toothache
Recommended forms: fresh/dried fruits in cooking; 10–20 drops Tabasco sauce in glass of water daily; tincture; freeze-dried extract; for topical use apply creams containing capsaicin (the active ingredient) up to six times daily

CAUTION External application may cause dermatitis. Do not touch eyes when handling fresh plants.

Cichorium intybus CHICORY

Part used: root
Properties: diuretic; digestive aid; laxative
Use for: fluid retention; constipation; bowel disorders (bloating, rumbling, etcetera)
Recommended form: powder (Use as an instant drink.)

Cimicifuga racemosa BLACK COHOSH

Part used: root
Properties: antispasmodic; oestrogen balancing
Use for: menopause; PMS; menstrual cramps
Recommended forms: tincture; standardized extract; freeze-dried extract

CAUTION Avoid in pregnancy.

Cinnamomum zeylanicum CINNAMON

Parts used: bark and twigs
Properties: carminative; vasodilator
Use for: indigestion; flatulence; circulation problems (such as chilblains or Raynaud's disease); high blood pressure
Recommended forms: decoction; powdered bark in food and drinks

Crataegus oxyacantha HAWTHORN

Parts used: berries and flowering tops
Properties: regulates heart rate; vasodilator; diuretic; anti-oxidant
Use for: cardiovascular disease; high blood pressure; fluid retention
Recommended forms: tincture; freeze-dried extract

Curcuma longa TURMERIC

Part used: root
Properties: potent antioxidant; anti-inflammatory; antimutagenic; antiviral
Use for: all painful inflammatory conditions (such as rheumatoid arthritis); ulcerative colitis; tissue injuries; cancer; AIDS
Recommended forms: extracts standardized for curcumin are recommended; freeze-dried extract

Echinacea purpurea/angustifolia ECHINACEA

Part used: root
Properties: immune stimulant; antimicrobial; anti-inflammatory; healing
Use for: all infections; depressed immune function; inflammatory conditions; allergies
Recommended forms: tincture; freeze-dried extract; cream for topical application
Note: Do not use continuously: echinacea preparations are more effective if taken one week on, one week off.

Eleutherococcus senticosus SIBERIAN GINSENG

Part used: root
Properties: increases endurance and resistance to stress; adaptogen
Use for: stress; nervous exhaustion; fatigue
Recommended forms: standardized or freeze-dried extract

Eschscholzia californica CALIFORNIAN POPPY

Parts used: aerial parts
Properties: sedative
Use for: anxiety; tension headaches; insomnia
Recommended forms: infusion; tincture

Foeniculum vulgare FENNEL

Part used: seed
Properties: carminative; antispasmodic; stimulates milk flow in nursing mothers
Use for: indigestion; colic; flatulence; insufficient breastmilk
Recommended forms: decoction; chew ½ tsp seeds after meals

Gingko biloba GINGKO/MAIDENHAIR TREE

Part used: leaf
Properties: powerful antioxidant; stimulates cardio-vascular, glandular and central nervous systems; immune stimulant; anti-allergic
Use for: age-related degenerative conditions; arterial insufficiency; Alzheimer's disease; short-term memory loss; reduced mental function; tinnitus; degenerative eye complaints; cardiovascular disease; asthma
Recommended forms: standardized or freeze-dried extract

Glycyrrhiza glabra LIQUORICE

Part used: roots
Properties: soothing; healing; expectorant; antiviral; anti-inflammatory; antispasmodic; antioxidant; immune stimulant
Use for: coughs; bronchitis; asthma; stomach ulcers; peptic ulcers; colic
Recommended forms: tincture; freeze-dried extract; deglycyrrhizinated liquorice (DGL) tablets for long-term ulcer treatment

CAUTION Avoid excessive or long-term use.
Avoid in pregnancy.
Avoid if you are using drugs such as digoxin.

Hamamelis virginiana WITCH HAZEL

Parts used: bark and leaves
Properties: anti-inflammatory; astringent; healing
Use for: sunburn; minor thermal burns; insect bites; bruises; varicose veins; haemorrhoids; to staunch bleeding wounds
Recommended form: cold distilled witch hazel (dilute 1:1 with water if it stings)

CAUTION Never take internally.

Hydrastis canadensis GOLDEN SEAL

Part used: root
Properties: antimicrobial; anti-inflammatory
Use for: gastrointestinal and respiratory problems; psoriasis; eczema; candidiasis; thrush; tonsillitis; gum disease; wounds
Recommended forms: powdered root capsules (sprinkle powder from capsules into wounds; mix 1 tsp powder with 2 cups hot water, strain, and use for gargling or douching)

CAUTION Avoid in pregnancy.
Avoid if you suffer from high blood pressure.

Hypericum perforatum ST JOHN'S WORT

Parts used: aerial parts
Properties: antidepressant; antiviral; anti-inflammatory; antispasmodic
Use for: depression; anxiety; emotional upsets; viral infections; insomnia; irritable bowel syndrome; burns; wounds; inflamed joints
Recommended forms: tincture; standardized extract; freeze-dried extract; cream or oil (for topical applications)

CAUTION Prolonged use may lead to photosensitivity.

Lavandula angustifolia LAVENDER

Part used: flower
Properties: sedative; anti-inflammatory; analgesic
Use for: insomnia; nervous tension; migraines; headaches
Recommended forms: infusion; tincture

CAUTION Avoid high doses in pregnancy.

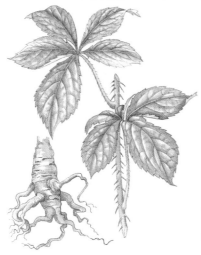

SIBERIAN GINSENG

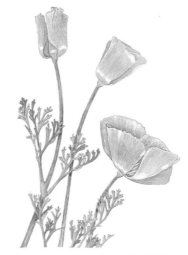

CALIFORNIAN POPPY

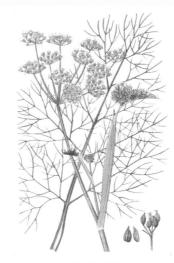

FENNEL

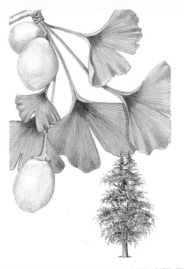

GINGKO/MAIDENHAIR TREE

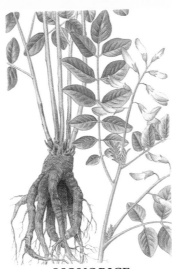

LIQUORICE

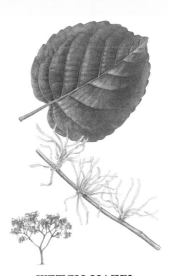

WITCH HAZEL

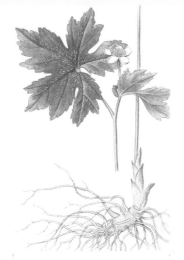

GOLDEN SEAL

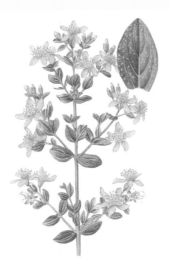

ST JOHN'S WORT

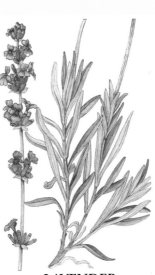

LAVENDER

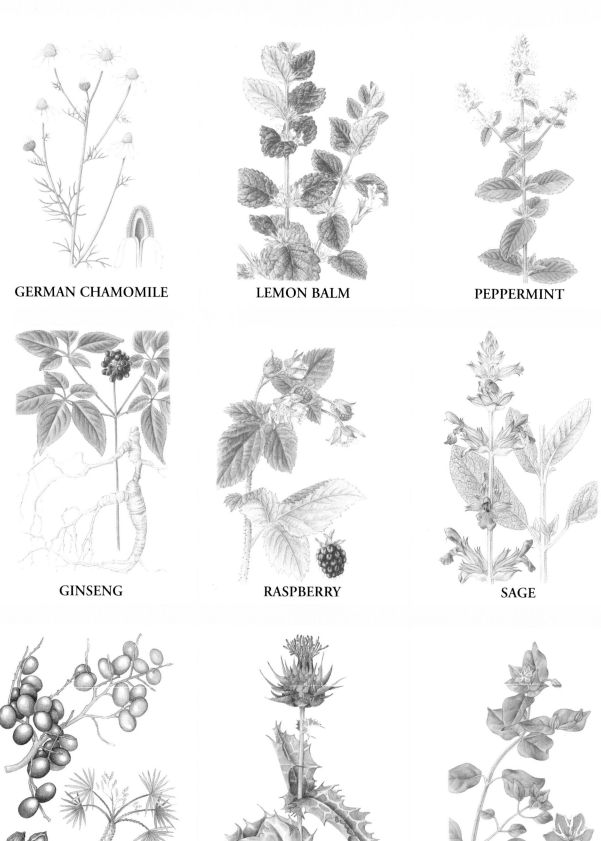

GERMAN CHAMOMILE

LEMON BALM

PEPPERMINT

GINSENG

RASPBERRY

SAGE

SAW PALMETTO

MILK THISTLE

CHICKWEED

Matricaria recutita **GERMAN CHAMOMILE**
Part used: flower
Properties: carminative; sedative; antispasmodic; immune stimulant
Use for: indigestion; colic; diarrhoea; teething; earache; insomnia; nervous upsets
Recommended form: infusion
Note: Roman chamomile *(Chamaemelum nobile)* has similar properties and uses.

Melissa officinalis **LEMON BALM**
Part used: leaf
Properties: antidepressant; sedative
Use for: depression; anxiety; tension headaches; nervous digestive upsets; indigestion
Recommended form: infusion

Mentha piperita **PEPPERMINT**
Part used: leaf
Properties: carminative; antispasmodic; central nervous system stimulant
Use for: nausea; migraine; heartburn; indigestion; colic; flatulence; irritable bowel syndrome (IBS); to improve alertness and concentration
Recommended forms: infusion; tincture; enteric-coated peppermint oil capsules for IBS

CAUTION   May reduce milk flow during breastfeeding.

Panax ginseng/P. quinquefolium **GINSENG**
Part used: root
Properties: invigorating; aphrodisiac; increases endurance, mood and resistance to stress; antioxidant; lowers cholesterol; regulates blood sugar; adaptogen
Use for: mental and physical exhaustion; cardiovascular disease; diabetes
Recommended form: standardized extract only

CAUTION   Long-term use may increase blood pressure. Avoid high doses in pregnancy.

Rubus idaeus **RASPBERRY**
Part used: leaf
Properties: astringent; antispasmodic; uterine tonic
Use for: diarrhoea; labour pains; menstrual cramps
Recommended form: infusion

CAUTION   Avoid in first seven months of pregnancy.

Salvia officinalis **SAGE**
Parts used: aerial parts
Properties: antimicrobial; oestrogen balancing
Use for: sore throats; gum infections; mouth ulcers; menstrual problems; menopause
Recommended forms: infusion (for gargle or mouth wash); tincture
Note: Red sage is the most medicinal type.

CAUTION   Avoid in pregnancy.

Serenoa repens **SAW PALMETTO**
Part used: berry
Properties: immune stimulant; diuretic; male aphrodisiac
Use for: benign prostatic hypertrophy; prostatitis; loss of libido
Recommended forms: standardized extract; freeze-dried extract

Silybum marianum **MILK THISTLE**
Parts used: aerial parts
Properties: powerful antioxidant; liver restorative and stimulant
Use for: hepatitis; cirrhosis of liver; hangover
Recommended forms: standardized extract; freeze-dried extract; tincture

Stachys betonica **WOOD BETONY**
Parts used: aerial parts *(not illustrated)*
Properties: sedative; vasodilator; analgesic
Use for: indigestion; headaches; migraines; gout; general aches and pains; anxiety; nervous tension
Recommended forms: infusion; tincture

CAUTION   Avoid high doses in pregnancy.

Stellaria media **CHICKWEED**
Parts used: aerial parts
Properties: healing; anti-inflammatory; astringent
Use for: eczema; boils; carbuncles; insect stings; splinters
Recommended forms: cream; infusion or tincture

Tanacetum parthenium FEVERFEW

Part used: leaf

Properties: analgesic; anti-inflammatory; anticoagulant

Use for: migraines; rheumatoid arthritis

Recommended forms: standardized extract; freeze-dried extract; fresh leaves

> **CAUTION** Avoid in pregnancy.
> Avoid if you are using anticoagulant drugs.

Taraxacum officinale DANDELION

Parts used: leaf; root

Properties: leaf acts as diuretic and is iron-rich; root acts as liver stimulant

Use leaf for: fluid retention; high blood pressure; anaemia

Use root for: skin and arthritic complaints

Recommended forms: freeze-dried extract; fresh leaves; powdered root

Tilia europaea LIME BLOSSOM/LINDEN

Part used: flower *(not illustrated)*

Properties: sedative; lowers blood pressure; reduces atherosclerosis; antioxidant

Use for: nervous tension; stress; tension headaches; cardiovascular disease; high blood pressure

Recommended forms: infusion; tincture

Ulmus rubra SLIPPERY ELM

Part used: inner bark

Properties: soothing; healing

Use for: sore throats; all digestive problems including gastritis, stomach ulcers and peptic ulcers; boils; abscesses

Recommended forms: tablets as directed; or mix 1 tsp powder with 250 ml (1 cup) boiling water, flavour with honey* and sip, repeating twice daily; or mix powder with hot water to make a warm poultice and apply to boil/abscess

*Use pasteurized honey for infants under one year old.

Urtica dioica STINGING NETTLE

Part used: leaf

Properties: anti-allergic; mineral-rich

Use for: hayfever; asthma; eczema; urticaria; anaemia; as nutritional supplement

Recommended forms: freeze-dried extract; infusion

Vaccinium myrtillus BILBERRY/BLUEBERRY

Part used: fruit

Properties: powerful antioxidant; improves blood flow to eyes; protects against cataracts and deteriorating vision

Use for: all eye problems

Recommended forms: standardized extract; freeze-dried extract

Verbena officinalis VERVAIN

Parts used: aerial parts

Properties: sedative; antidepressant

Use for: anxiety; depression

Recommended forms: infusion; tincture

> **CAUTION** Avoid high doses in pregnancy.

Viburnum opulus GUELDER ROSE/ CRAMP BARK

Part used: bark

Properties: antispasmodic; anti-inflammatory; sedative

Use for: menstrual cramps; irritable bowel syndrome; muscle cramps

Recommended forms: tincture; freeze-dried extract

Vitex agnus-castus CHASTE TREE/ AGNUS CASTUS

Part used: berry

Properties: oestrogen balancing

Use for: menstrual problems; menopause

Recommended forms: tincture; freeze-dried extract

> **CAUTION** Avoid in pregnancy.

Zingiber officinalis GINGER

Part used: root

Properties: antioxidant; carminative; anti-inflammatory; anticoagulant; reduces blood pressure and cholesterol levels; vasodilator

Use for: indigestion; nausea; inflammatory conditions (such as rheumatoid arthritis or ulcerative colitis); cardiovascular disease; high blood pressure; hiccups

Recommended forms: 1 tsp grated fresh root in food or drink three times daily; tincture; capsules

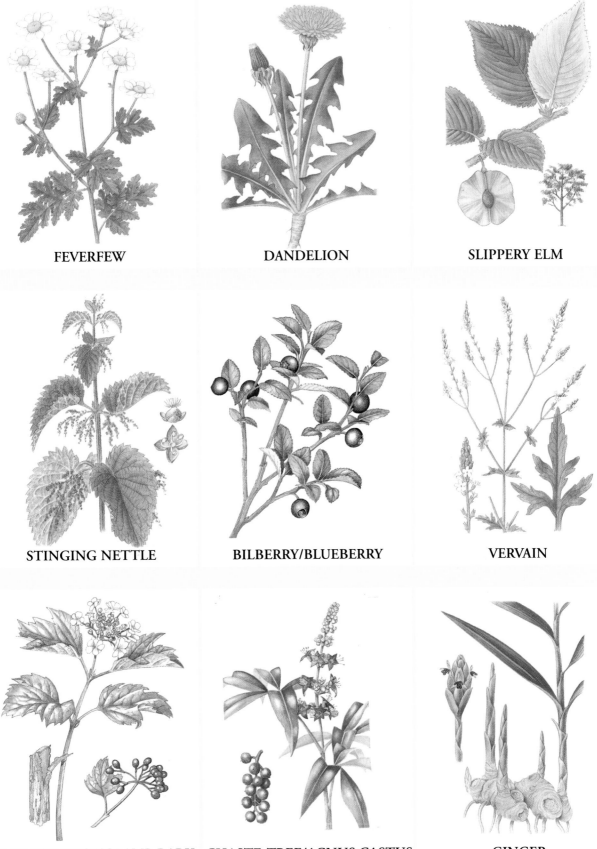

FEVERFEW

DANDELION

SLIPPERY ELM

STINGING NETTLE

BILBERRY/BLUEBERRY

VERVAIN

GUELDER ROSE/CRAMP BARK

CHASTE TREE/AGNUS CASTUS

GINGER

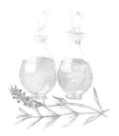

AROMATHERAPY

Aromatherapy is a modern term for the ancient practice of using essential oils extracted from aromatic herbs to enhance health and happiness. Essential oils have a two-fold effect: an internal, physiological one and an emotional one. This makes them a fascinating, pleasurable and effective addition to the natural home pharmacy.

HOW THE ESSENTIAL OILS WORK

Essential oils are produced by aromatic plants partly as a defence mechanism, so it is not surprising that some of their chemical constituents have been found to be powerful antibacterial, antifungal and anti-viral substances. Research into the effects of the main active ingredients has revealed many other therapeutic properties, ranging from analgesic and sedative to antispasmodic and anti-inflammatory properties. Essential oils also have an

Above: It takes roughly 70 kg (154 lb) of plant material to produce 2 litres (3½ pints) of essential oil. Some oils are expensive because of the amount of raw material required: it takes 200 kg (440 lb) of rose petals to produce 1 litre (1¾ pints) of rose essential oil.

effect on the central nervous system, especially the brain. (For example, lavender oil has a sedative and calming effect, while rosemary oil has a stimulating effect, improving alertness.)

The volatile aromatic substances are absorbed either through the skin or the lungs. From there they enter the body tissues and bloodstream, bringing about widespread effects throughout the body. (Some of the chemicals can be skin irritants, which is why they should always be used in a diluted form.)

There is, however, another subtle, much more complex effect of aromatherapy, and that is the emotional response to smell itself. Aroma molecules travel up the nose to receptor sites on the olfactory bulbs. From there messages are sent directly to the limbic system, the so-called 'primitive' brain, which deals with emotions, mood, arousal and memory. Some smells, such as the scent of roses, are found universally pleasing and usually evoke positive emotions. Other odours, such as that of rotten eggs, are repulsive and will bring on negative emotions and even nausea. Most smells, however, have a unique and highly personal emotional effect dependent on the person's past associations. (A particular perfume might bring back a flood of sad memories to someone who has lost a friend who used to wear it. The same perfume might sexually arouse another if their partner wears it.) This is why it is extremely important in aromatherapy to choose essential oils that appeal to you. You can then build on the pleasant associations by using the appropriate oil in a deep-relaxing massage or your bath. Eventually you'll find that the smell alone will bring about all the emotional and physical benefits that the original massage or long soak induced. This is known as an aroma-conditioned reflex.

HOW TO USE THE ESSENTIAL OILS

There are several ways to use essential oils: in combination with a massage, on a compress, in the bath, in a steam inhalation or by inhaling directly from a handkerchief. First choose oils with the required properties. These oils can be used singly or in combinations of up to three at a time. Try to select and/or blend oils which are pleasing to the person being treated. If a carrier oil is recommended, use one of the following: sweet almond oil, sunflower oil, soya oil, olive oil or apricot kernel oil.

AROMA-CONDITIONED REFLEX

Experiments are revealing wide applications for aroma-conditioned reflexes. Odours can, through association, be used to depress or stimulate appetites, induce relaxation and sleep and improve memory. Odour memories can be powerful and long lasting: sometimes just a whiff of a smell familiar from childhood can bring back strong memories and emotions from that time.

Right: *Use a range of delightful aromatherapy oils in your bath to positively influence your mood and, in the long term, your health. To lift depression use bergamot, geranium, melissa, jasmine or rose oil; to calm and soothe use lavender, neroli, sandalwood or ylang ylang; for mental fatigue use peppermint or rosemary oil.*

CAUTION

- It is recommended that all oils are avoided during the first three months of pregnancy, unless professionally prescribed.
- Purchase pure, unadulterated essential oils from reputable companies only.
- Don't apply undiluted oils to the skin unless you have been specifically directed to do so.
- Do a patch test first to check for sensitivity: apply a normal dilution of oil to the inside of your elbow, cover with a plaster and examine after two hours. If there is any redness or itching, do not use that oil.
- Never take the oils internally unless under professional supervision.
- Avoid prolonged use of the same oil.
- Keep essential oils away from eyes and from children.
- Label bottles clearly with name, dilution and date, and store in a cool, dark place.

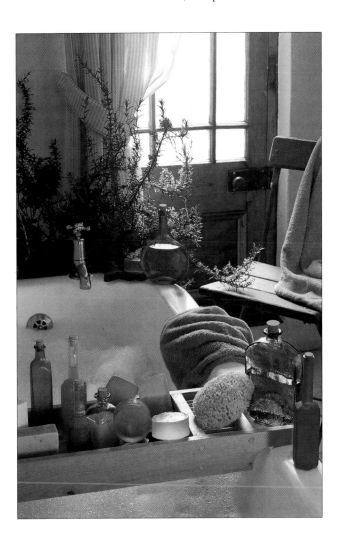

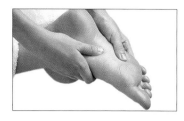

For a massage

Mix a total of 10 drops essential oil/s with 20 ml (2 tbsp) carrier oil. For a smaller quantity, add 2–3 drops essential oil to 5 ml (1 tsp) carrier oil. For young children and sensitive skins, use up to 5 drops per 20 ml (2 tbsp) carrier oil. Use these dilutions with the massage techniques recommended on pp. 74–77.

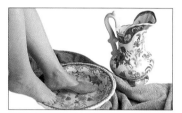

For a bath

Add 5–10 drops essential oil to a warm bath, lie back, relax and breathe deeply. A smaller foot bath using 5 drops essential oil can also be used.

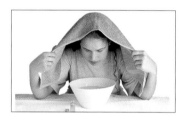

Steam inhalation

Add 2–3 drops essential oil to a basin of hot water. Lean over the basin, cover your head with a towel and breathe in deeply through your nose for up to 10 minutes. Repeat three times a day for acute conditions such as chest infections, colds, coughs and sinusitis. Do not use for treating asthma, or if you have a sensitive skin.

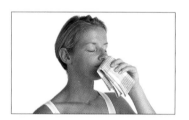

Direct inhalation

Place 2–3 drops on a handkerchief, hold close to the nose and inhale deeply. At night, a treated handkerchief can be placed on the pillow near the nose. Alternatively, use a vaporizer.

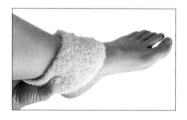

Compresses

Use warm compresses for muscular aches and pains, abdominal cramps, toothache, boils and abscesses; use cold compresses for bruises, sprains, swollen joints, inflammation and headaches. Add 5 drops essential oil to 1 litre (1¾ pints) hot or cold water and mix. Soak a cloth in the mixture, wring out and place on affected area. Re-soak cloth when compress reaches body temperature. Repeat for up to 20 minutes.

SOME USEFUL ESSENTIAL OILS FOR THE HOME PHARMACY

CYPRESS (*Cupressus sempervirens*)
Parts used: needles and twigs
Properties: anti-inflammatory; anti-spasmodic; astringent
Use for: bronchitis; coughs; asthma; rheumatic aches and pains; haemorrhoids; broken capillaries; bruises; varicose veins; skin toner (good for oily skin); sweaty feet

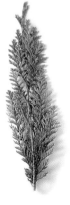

SANDALWOOD (*Santalum album*)
Part used: wood
Properties: sedative; antibacterial; anti-inflammatory
Use for: stress-related mental disorders (anxiety, depression, insomnia, etcetera); bronchitis; sore throats; laryngitis; acne; eczema; dry, sensitive skin

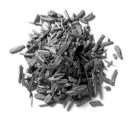

CHAMOMILE (Use either Roman chamomile [*Chamaemelum nobile/Anthemis nobilis*] or German chamomile [*Matricaria recutita*]; both have similar properties, although the Roman chamomile appears to have stronger sedative properties while German chamomile is more anti-inflammatory and analgesic.)

Part used: flower

Properties: sedative; analgesic; anti-inflammatory; antispasmodic; carminative

Use for: stress-related mental disorders (anxiety, depression, insomnia, irritability and nervous tension); painful dentition; tension headaches; muscular aches, pains and swollen joints; colic; indigestion and flatulence; irritable bowel syndrome; eczema; dry, chapped skin; psoriasis; urticaria; dermatitis

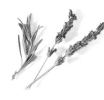

LAVENDER (*Lavandula angustifolia/officinalis*)

Parts used: flowering tops

Properties: sedative; analgesic; antibacterial; antispasmodic; insecticide

Use for: stress-related mental disorders (anxiety, depression, grief, insomnia, etcetera); headaches and migraines; rheumatic aches and pains; indigestion; colic and flatulence; pimples and spots; wounds; burns; bruises; insect bites and stings; to rid someone of lice, fleas and mites

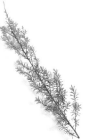

TEA TREE (*Melaleuca alternifolia*)

Part used: leaf

Properties: antibacterial; antifungal; antiviral; decongestant; insecticide

Use for: bronchitis; coughs; sore throats; sinusitis; acne; thrush; athlete's foot; ringworm; dandruff; herpes; wounds; cuts; insect stings and bites; to rid someone of lice (nits) and mites

GERANIUM (*Pelargonium graveolens*)

Parts used: whole plant

Properties: antidepressant; antibacterial; antifungal; astringent; insecticide (similar function to rose oil but much cheaper)

Use for: stress-related disorders; thrush; wounds (will stop bleeding); various skin problems (including haemorrhoids, broken capillaries, bruises, varicose veins); good skin toner; insect repellant

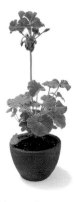

CAUTION May cause skin irritation, so should be used in lower dilutions – 5 drops to 2 tbsp carrier oil.

ROSEMARY (*Rosmarinus officinalis*)

Parts used: flowering tops

Properties: mental and circulatory system stimulant; analgesic; anti-inflammatory; astringent

Use for: mental and physical exhaustion; failing memory; headaches; arthritis; rheumatism; skin toner; hair conditioner; dandruff

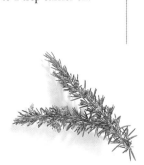

CLARY SAGE (*Salvia sclarea*)

Parts used: flowering tops

Properties: sedative; analgesic; anti-inflammatory; antispasmodic; oestrogen balancing; hormone regulator.

Use for: stress-related mental disorders (anxiety, depression, insomnia, etcetera); sore throats; menstrual problems, especially period pains and PMS

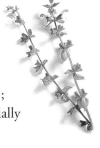

CAUTION Avoid in pregnancy.

EUCALYPTUS (*Eucalyptus globulus*)

Part used: leaf

Properties: analgesic; antibacterial; antiviral; anti-inflammatory; expectorant

Use for: colds; flu; bronchitis; sinusitis; asthma; rheumatic aches and pains; wounds; skin ulcers; herpes

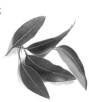

CAUTION May cause skin irritation, so should be used in lower dilutions – 5 drops to 20 ml (2 tbsp) carrier oil.

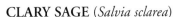

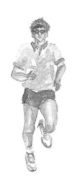

EXERCISE

Movement is a fundamental aspect of life itself, so it is not surprising that activity confers vital benefits and that inactivity compromises health. The lives of adults and children have become increasingly sedentary as the usual opportunities for everyday exercise have been eroded by our reliance on technology to transport and entertain us. Inactivity is now implicated in so many of the chronic degenerative and mental ailments that plague the developed world so it is no longer possible to ignore exercise as a basic requirement for good health. Exercise is thus one of the first therapies one should try.

Above: *Aerobic exercise increases the production of human growth hormone, also known as anti-ageing hormone. This hormone, the production of which declines rapidly with age, increases energy levels, sexual performance, immune response, bone density and muscle mass. It also elevates mood, sharpens vision, stimulates hair growth and leads to a smoother, firmer skin.*

WHAT KIND OF EXERCISE?

There are two basic kinds of exercise: aerobic and non-aerobic. Aerobic exercise, the more beneficial type, describes any activity that substantially increases your heart and respiratory rate and improves your cardiovascular fitness. It should never lead to serious discomfort, to pain or to extreme breathlessness (you should just be able to hold a conversation while doing any kind of aerobic exercise). Non-aerobic types of exercise (such as yoga or weight training) do not usually increase your heart and breathing rate to any significant degree, but confer other benefits, such as an improvement in joint flexibility and muscle strength.

AEROBIC ACTIVITIES

The following information is provided to help you choose a suitable aerobic exercise programme. Remember to vary the activity, and that every bit of aerobic exercise helps; daily activities such as housework, gardening and climbing stairs can easily qualify as aerobic exercise if they are performed with vigour!

WALKING One of the best and safest activities. However, a frequent problem is that walking is not done strenuously enough to qualify as aerobic. A speed of 6–8 km/h (4–5 miles/h) should be maintained on the flat for at least 30 minutes.

RUNNING This is excellent for building up strength, stamina and fitness, but the chances of injury are high, especially to the back, hip, knee and ankle joints. Avoid very hard running surfaces such as concrete and tarmac.

DANCING This is a most underrated and beneficial form of exercise. All types of dancing, from classical to country, offer excellent advantages for aerobic activity and have the added advantage of being highly enjoyable.

SKIPPING An often overlooked but excellent aerobic exercise, which can be done anywhere as long as you have a skipping rope.

AEROBICS Aerobics classes are good for people who have trouble motivating themselves. However, many of the high-impact activities can traumatize joints, and low-impact aerobics classes are more suitable for beginners.

SWIMMING This is the activity of choice for all people with musculoskeletal problems such as arthritis. Water supports the body and, by removing the stress of gravity, allows for freer movement of the joints and muscles. If you don't like swimming lengths, join an aqua aerobics class. (Note: swimming is not a weight-bearing activity and therefore does not increase bone density.)

CYCLING Speeds of no less than 15 km/h (10 miles/h) on the flat should be maintained. Stationary exercise bicycles can be used.

Many other sports and activities offer chances for aerobic exercise, the most beneficial ones being those that require sustained activity (such as canoeing or cross-country skiing) rather than 'stop-start' games (such as tennis).

How to begin

Firstly it's necessary to establish your state of fitness so that you understand your limits and have a yardstick by which to measure your progress. Your pulse rate (the number of times your heart beats) while you are resting reflects your level of fitness. As you begin to exercise regularly two things happen:

1 Your blood carries more oxygen because of an improved oxygen/carbon dioxide exchange in your lungs.

2 Your muscles use the oxygen more effectively.

The overall result of this improved efficiency is that less blood is required to do the same amount of work, so your heart slows down. This is the effect you should aim to achieve.

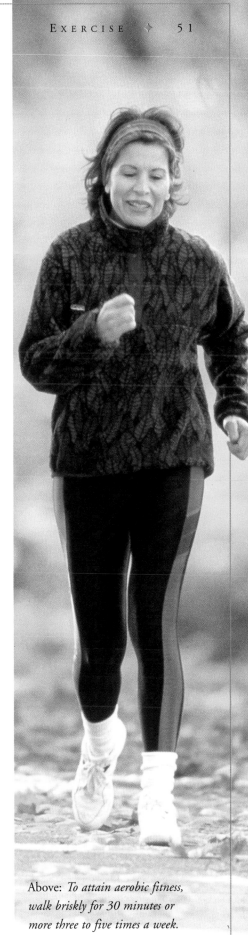

Above: *To attain aerobic fitness, walk briskly for 30 minutes or more three to five times a week.*

THE BENEFITS OF AEROBIC EXERCISE

- Improves mental state and mood. Exercise has been found to be as effective as psychotherapy in the treatment of mild/moderate depression.
- Improves energy levels and overall sense of wellbeing.
- Improves sleeping habits.
- Decreases tension.
- Lowers cholesterol levels. Exercise lowers the harmful LDL cholesterol levels but raises the beneficial HDL levels (p. 15).
- Lowers blood pressure.
- Improves circulation and the movement of lymph – important for getting nutrients to and waste from body tissues.
- Increases strength, function and tone of muscles, including the heart.
- Increases joint flexibility and strength and improves sense of balance – important for the elderly who are more likely to fall.
- Increases respiratory capacity and lung function.
- Improves digestion and bowel transit time, substantially reducing the risk of colon cancer.
- Improves immune function.
- Decreases body fat and increases metabolic rate, preventing and treating obesity.
- Improves skin condition.

- Slows down the loss of calcium from bones, reducing the risk of osteoporosis and bone fractures.
- Stabilizes blood sugar levels, reducing the incidence of diabetes and hypoglycaemia.
- Normalizes oestrogen production, reducing the incidence of menstrual disorders and breast, uterine and cervical cancer.
- Decreases overall mortality, especially from cardiovascular disease.

NOTE:

It is not necessary to adopt a vigorous training schedule to experience these benefits. All that is required is 20–30 minutes of aerobic exercise three to five days a week. If we don't exercise the maxim 'what we don't use we lose' applies, and the converse of all these benefits happens. Muscles become weak and start to degenerate, joints stiffen, ligaments tighten and bones become soft due to calcium loss.

It is possible to have too much of a good thing: while regular moderate to vigorous exercise improves the immune response, too much exercise may compromise it. Marathon runners know that they have to be careful after a race as they are much more prone to infections. Similarly, female athletes who overdo their training programmes can reduce the production of oestrogen to such an extent that they stop menstruating. If this state continues for any length of time it may adversely affect the deposition of calcium in their bones, making them more vulnerable to osteoporosis in later life.

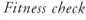

Fitness check

Measure your pulse rate first thing in the morning while you are still in bed. Make sure you have a watch which displays seconds. Place the first two fingers of your left hand on your right wrist just below the base of your thumb. Don't press too hard. Once you have located your pulse, count the number of beats per minute. As you become familiar with the procedure you can do a quick assessment by counting the number of beats in 10 seconds and multiplying by six. During exercise, stop briefly and check your pulse rate immediately. It should not rise above 80% of the maximum rate for your age (see opposite). If it does, slow down and take frequent breaks.

TRAINING ZONE IN HEARTBEATS PER MINUTE

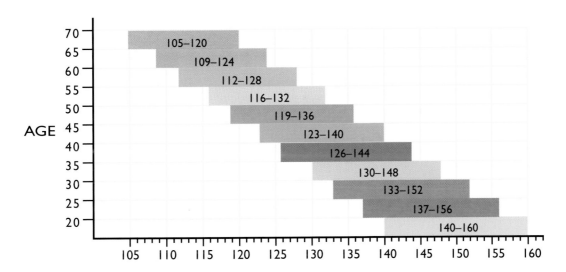

Training effect

To ensure that the type of exercise you are doing is having a 'training effect', your pulse rate must rise sufficiently, (in other words, your pulse rate should reach between 70–80% of the maximum pulse rate (MPR) for your age). To calculate this figure, subtract your age from 220. Then multiply by 70% or 80%.

Example

220 – 40 years old = 180 MPR
180 x 70% = 126 beats/minute
180 x 80% = 144 beats/minute
The 'training effect' will therefore occur between 126 and 144 beats per minute.

Recovery rate

The rate at which your pulse is restored to its resting level is a very good measure of fitness. Take your pulse rate at intervals of one, five and ten minutes after the exercise. If it is still raised after ten minutes, then the activity is too strenuous and it should be moderated.

FITNESS LEVEL (HEARTBEATS PER MINUTE)

AGE	VERY FIT	FIT	MODERATE	UNFIT
Men				
20–29	less than 60	60–69	70–85	over 85
30–39	less than 64	64–71	72–85	over 85
40–49	less than 65	65–73	74–90	over 90
50+	less than 68	68–75	76–90	over 90
Women				
20–29	less than 72	72–77	78–95	over 95
30–39	less than 72	72–79	80–97	over 97
40–49	less than 75	75–79	80–98	over 98
50+	less than 75	76–85	85–102	over 102

Note: These figures are general guides only: there is a fair variation in people's pulse rates owing to genetic factors. However, if you fall into the unfit category or are over 40 years old it is advisable to have a medical checkup before starting an exercise programme.

After a ten-week programme of regular exercise your pulse rate will have slowed down and become stronger. You will then have to exercise harder to achieve the training effect. However, by this stage you will want to do just that, as you will be experiencing all the beneficial effects mentioned previously.

Recommended programme

Choose activities which are pleasurable and suited to your age, state of health and temperament. Try to exercise at least three times a week for 30 minutes. Avoid competitive sports if you suffer from stress and tension. If you are just beginning an exercise programme you should either participate in organized classes or join up with others; people who exercise alone are more likely to give up or find excuses not to exercise. All types of exercise carry an injury risk, some more than others. Hip, knee and ankle joints are particularly vulnerable, as are muscles, tendons and ligaments. You are less likely to injure yourself or become sick if you observe the following advice:

1 Build up your level of fitness gradually – irregular and violent activity confers no benefits and may have serious medical repercussions. If you cannot manage 30 minutes of sustained aerobic exercise, break it up into manageable periods.

2 Warm up properly before strenuous exercise with a programme of stretching exercises (p. 55).

3 Stop and rest if you experience any sort of pain, discomfort or acute breathlessness.

4 Invest in the correct equipment, such as good training shoes for all running activities. Wear loose cotton clothes and cover up well after exercise.

5 Do not exercise when you are very tired, sick or feverish.

6 Do not exercise on a full stomach.

7 The benefits of exercise are enhanced if followed by a relaxation activity (pp. 83–84).

Exercise	Stamina	Strength	Flexibility	Coordination	Posture
AEROBIC					
Walking	***	*	*	*	*
Running	***	**	*	*	*
Dancing	***	**	**	***	**
Cycling	***	**	*	*	–
Swimming	***	**	**	**	*
NON-AEROBIC					
Yoga	*	*	***	**	***
Weights	*	***	–	**	*

KEY: Fair *   Good **   Excellent ***

NON-AEROBIC EXERCISE

Non-aerobic exercise offers some of the benefits of aerobic exercise, such as counteracting the effects of stress and improving joint flexibility and muscle tone. In some of these areas it can be superior to aerobic exercise.

YOGA These exercises offer a balanced series of stretching movements which increase the suppleness of the spine and improve overall flexibility, posture and general muscle tone. Yoga is an excellent stress reducer and aid to relaxation and is highly recommended for every age group.

WEIGHT TRAINING These are exercises which make the muscles work against resistance and are good for increasing muscle strength, tone and size as well as bone density.

ALL-ROUND FITNESS

Different types of exercise are good for different aspects of fitness: it is possible to gain strength and stamina without flexibility. If you cannot easily touch your toes while sitting with your legs stretched out in front of you, then you need to develop your flexibility as well as your fitness. We recommend a varied programme of aerobic exercise and the following sequence of yoga exercises, which should be practised daily (repeat three times) to promote spine suppleness and strength (p. 129), and as a pre-exercise warm-up. Try to follow the breathing sequence and to make the movements as flowing and relaxed as possible.

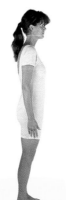

1

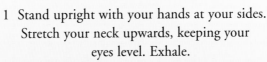

Salute to the Sun

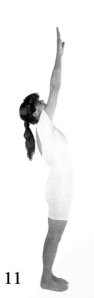

11

1 Stand upright with your hands at your sides.
Stretch your neck upwards, keeping your
eyes level. Exhale.

2 Inhale deeply as you raise your arms upwards and over your head, keeping your hands together. Bend back from the waist as far as is comfortable.

3 Exhale slowly as you bring your arms back over your head and bend over to
place your hands either side of your feet. Bring your face as close to your legs as
possible. Bend your knees if you have to.

4 Inhaling, bend your right knee up as you stretch your left leg back as illustrated.
Extend your neck and look up.

5 Hold your breath as you stretch your right leg back to join your left leg. Your
body should be straight, and supported by your toes and extended arms.

6 Exhale as you lower your knees, chest and forehead to the floor. Keep your stomach
and pelvis off the floor.

10

7 Inhale as you lower your stomach to the floor while extending your arms
to lift your chest up. Extend your neck and look up.

8 Lower your chest to the floor and then exhale as you tuck your toes
under and push your hips up as illustrated. Push your heels towards the ground.

9 Inhale as you bring your left leg forwards and under your chest.
Extend your neck and look up.

10 Exhale while you bring your right leg alongside your left. As you do this,
extend both legs, lifting your buttocks up but keeping your hands on the
ground and your face close to your legs.

11 Inhale as you straighten, lifting your arms up and over your head
again. Arch your back. Exhale as you return to your
original position, with hands by your sides.
When you have finished, adopt the corpse position
(p. 83) and practise the progressive muscle relaxation
routine (pp. 83–84) for five minutes.

2

3

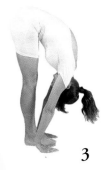

4

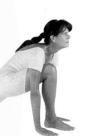

5

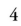

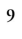
9

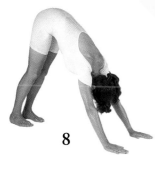
8

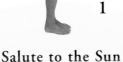
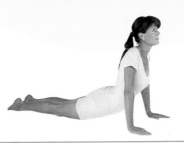
7

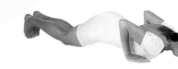
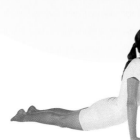
6

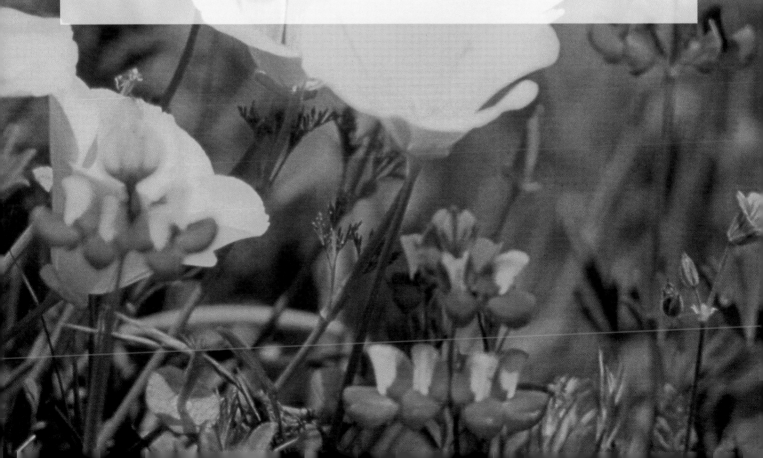

ENERGY REMEDIES

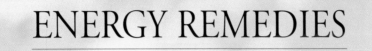

*A*dvanced physics has demonstrated that all matter is really energy vibrating at different frequencies. Life is therefore a complex network of interwoven energy fields. We are all familiar with the apparently dense matter of the physical human body, but are often unfamiliar with the more subtle, invisible energy fields which permeate and vitalise it. These energy fields are often referred to as the life force or etheric body; in Chinese medicine they are called Chi and in Ayurvedic medicine Prana.

Although homeopathic and flower remedies are made differently, they both use the subtle energy or vibrational imprint of a particular substance or flower to restore or balance our own subtle energy fields. This stimulates cellular activity, which brings about a healing response on an emotional and physical plane. Although it is not yet understood how this happens, numerous experiments show conclusively that water can retain a 'vibrational memory'. This vibrational imprint affects our subtle energy fields, which in turn stimulates a healing response on an emotional and physical level. This chapter explains how to select and use homeopathic and flower remedies in the treatment of disease and emotional disharmony.

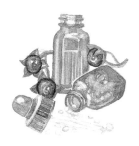

HOMEOPATHY

Homeopathy is a safe yet effective method of treating disease using specially diluted remedies. The homeopathic view sees symptoms of disease as signs of the body's attempt to heal itself, a process which should be gently encouraged, not counteracted. Homeopathic remedies are therefore selected according to their ability to replicate the symptoms of the illness and thus stimulate healing (using 'like to treat like'). For example, onion juice causes the nose to stream and the eyes to water. These are common hayfever symptoms, and a homeopathic remedy made from onion, Allium cepa, can be a very effective treatment for hayfever.

Although homeopathic remedies are extremely dilute, several clinical trials have demonstrated their effectiveness. Additional experiments have shown that homeopathic remedies have a stimulating and healing effect both on diseased or poisoned cells as well as on enzyme activity.

Above: *Samuel Hahnemann (1755–1843), a German doctor, developed homeopathy as a safe alternative to the use of harmful drugs.*

HOW TO USE HOMEOPATHIC REMEDIES

There are no contraindications for the use of homeopathy. It is totally safe and eminently suitable for the home pharmacy. No harm can come of prescribing the wrong remedy – it will simply be ineffective. A child can swallow a whole bottleful of tablets without ill effect. All remedies should be taken between meals on a clean tongue – that is, without food or liquid.

Homeopathic remedies are available in two different dilution ranges: the centesimal range (denoted by a C) and the decimal range (denoted by an X). Although there are many different dilutions or potencies available, the most commonly used are 6X, 6C, 30C, 200C and 1M (1000C). The higher potencies are not necessarily more effective than the lower potencies. Some commercial preparations mix together different potencies of the same remedy.

While there are no hard-and-fast rules, the following guidelines are suggested:

- 30C is effective for a wide range of conditions. 6C is usually used for chronic, long-term problems. Alternatively, use a multi-potency remedy.
- Infants, children, adults and the elderly all receive the same dose. **Homeopathy is not dose dependent** (doubling the dosage will not double its effectiveness). It is the frequency of administration which is of greater importance.
- One tablet/pillule should be dissolved under the tongue, where it is quickly absorbed. For babies, crush a tablet between two spoons and drop the powder in the mouth.
- In cases of lactose intolerance (the pills are made with lactose), request a liquid preparation and take a couple of drops under the tongue.
- Occasionally a temporary worsening of symptoms is experienced, but persevere if this happens.

DOSAGE

For acute symptoms and emergencies dose every 10 minutes until there is an improvement. Then reduce the frequency to every 2 hours and stop once the patient shows strong signs of recovery. Less intense acute conditions can be treated every 2–4 hours. Homeopathic remedies work very quickly in acute problems; if there is no improvement within 2–3 hours, change the remedy. **For chronic conditions** dose three times daily until there is an improvement. If no improvement is experienced within 2–3 weeks, change the remedy.

HOW TO CHOOSE THE CORRECT REMEDIES

Homeopathy is a holistic discipline and the whole person is seen to be important: both the mental and the physical manifestations of a disease must be considered when choosing a remedy.

On the following pages we have listed the conditions the remedies can treat, followed by 'keynotes'. Any illness which is characterized by certain keynotes should respond to that remedy. In fact, the keynotes often take precedence over the symptoms of illness: for example, Belladonna is useful in a wide variety of infections and fevers, but so are Aconite, Bryonia and Hepar sulph. However, when selecting the remedy identify at least one of the keynotes: a fever character-ized by a **throbbing** headache and a **flushed** face would suggest Belladonna, while one characterized by **restlessness** and **anxiety** would suggest Aconite.

Homeopathic remedies are an ideal first-line treatment; however, if symptoms don't improve it is essential to consult a qualified practitioner. The remedies overleaf have such a wide sphere of action that they are an essential part of the home pharmacy.

BIOCHEMIC TISSUE SALTS

This range of twelve homeopathic remedies (6X) made from mineral salts was carefully selected by Dr W. Schuessler, a German homeopathic physician, as being important to health and specifically indicated to treat a variety of common ailments. They are used singly or in specific combinations to treat a variety of symptoms. Biochemic tissue salts are freely available and come with indications for their use.

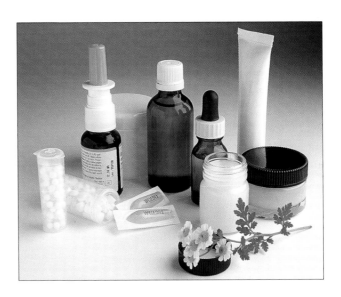

Above: *Homeopathic remedies come in powder, pillule/tablet or liquid form. Many of the remedies are also available as creams, ointments, nasal sprays and suppositories. Useful creams and ointments include Arnica, Hamamelis, Hypericum, Graphites and Urtica urens.*

RECOMMENDED REMEDIES FOR THE HOME PHARMACY

ACONITE
Use for: all fevers; colds; sore throats; croup; coughs; panic attacks; asthma; mental or physical shock; fright
Keynotes:
- symptoms come on suddenly, often after exposure to cold, dry winds
- fear/panic/anxiety
- extreme restlessness and thirst
- dry, suffocating cough

ARNICA
Use for: any injuries or accidents; any surgery or dental work; bruises; sprains; concussion; childbirth; aches and pains following physical exertion; insomnia
Keynotes:
- all mental and physical shock and trauma
- bed feels too hard

ARSENICUM ALBUM
Use for: gastrointestinal upsets including vomiting and diarrhoea; food poisoning; asthma; hayfever; colds; flu; anxiety; psoriasis; boils
Keynotes:
- chilly
- restless and irritable
- extreme exhaustion, out of all proportion to the complaint
- fearful, especially about the condition

- burning sensation in all parts
- worse around midnight
- relieved by warmth

BELLADONNA
Use for: fevers; chicken pox; measles; mumps; sore throats; toothache; inflammations; earache; boils; headaches; heatstroke
Keynotes:
- symptoms sudden and intense
- throbbing pains
- flushed face and hot, burning, dry skin
- dilated pupils
- confusion through to delirium
- worsens with noise, touch and lying down
- improves when erect

BRYONIA
Use for: coughs; colds; flu; laryngitis; bronchitis; headaches; joint pains; rheumatism
Keynotes:
- symptoms worsen with movement
- dryness of all mucous membranes (nose, mouth and lungs)
- great thirst
- improves on application of cold compress and with firm pressure
- worse with heat and in warm rooms

CHAMOMILLA
(excellent for children)
Use for: colic; teething; earache; toothache; asthma
Keynotes:
- irritable and bad tempered
- hypersensitive to pain
- impatient and whining
- child wants to be carried constantly
- thirsty
Note: Mental calmness contraindicates this remedy.

FERRUM PHOS
Use for: initial stages of all fevers and infections
Keynotes:
- fatigue and malaise
- vague, ill-defined symptoms
- worse at night

GELSEMIUM
Use for: anxiety and nervousness preceding all tasks, both major and minor; colds; flu; headaches; measles
Keynotes:
- trembling
- dizziness
- nasal congestion with feeling of tight band around head
- muscular weakness and pain
- drooping, heavy eyes

NUX VOMICA
Use for: indigestion from overindulgence; nausea; vomiting; constipation (with much ineffectual urging); bloating and pain 2–3 hours after eating; hangovers; colds; headaches and migraine; asthma; measles
Keynotes:
- irritable, impatient and quarrelsome
- fault-finding
- hypersensitive to noise, smells and light

PULSATILLA
(ideal for a range of childhood complaints)
Use for: teething; eye and ear problems; mumps; chickenpox; asthma; menstrual complaints; bronchitis; coughs; sinusitis.
Keynotes:
- symptoms and moods always changing
- weepy and clinging
- gentle, sympathetic nature
- copious yellow-green discharge
- worse after eating rich, fatty foods
- better in cool air and with company
- little or no thirst

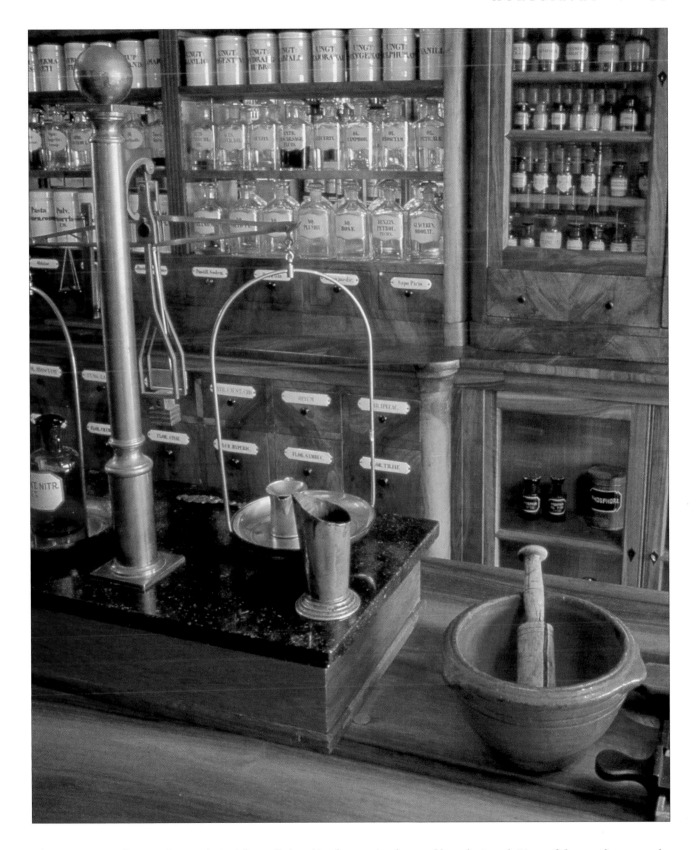

Above: *Homeopathic remedies are derived from all three kingdoms: animal, vegetable and mineral. Many of the remedies are made from the drugs that were used in Hahnemann's day (1755–1843), such as arsenic, mercury, belladonna and aconite. These drugs, which can be fatal in ordinary doses, have been shown to stimulate healing responses when taken in minute homeopathic doses.*

QUICK REFERENCE GUIDE TO OTHER USEFUL REMEDIES

As many commercial preparations contain a mixture of several remedies, this guide
will enable you to check their properties and indications.

REMEDY	USE FOR	KEYNOTES
ALLIUM CEPA	hayfever; conjunctivitis; colds	violent sneezing; burning discharges
APIS	tonsillitis; cystitis; insect bites	burning; stinging; swelling
ARGENTUM NITRICUM (ARG. NIT.)	mental exhaustion; anxiety preceding 'ordeals' such as exams or surgery; diarrhoea; bloating	nervousness; irrationality; fear; craving for sweet foods; trembling of limbs
BAPTISIA	all fevers and infections	muscular soreness; offensive secretions
CALC. FLUOR.	piles; varicose veins; scar tissue; adhesion	better with warmth
CANTHARIS	burns and scalds including sunburn; cystitis	hot, burning pains
COCCULUS	nausea; motion sickness; headaches; low back pain	extreme exhaustion; weakness and numbness; dizziness
COFFEA	insomnia due to mental activity and tension	restlessness; agitation; hypersensitivity
COLOCYNTHIS	nausea; vomiting; colic; diarrhoea; menstrual pains	irritability; violent cramping pains; better with pressure and when doubled over
CUPRUM	cramps; spasms; convulsions; whooping cough	violent symptoms
DIOSCOREA	abdominal pains and cramps; infant colic	sharp, twisting, shooting pains; worse when doubled over; better when stretched out
DROSERA	whooping cough; dry cough	retching; hoarseness
ECHINACEA	all fevers and septic conditions	fatigue; aching limbs
EUPATORIUM	colds; flu	deep bone pains
EUPHRASIA	conjunctivitis; eyestrain; colds; hayfever	copious burning, watery secretions
GRAPHITES	skin eruptions; keloids	itchy, oozing discharges
HAMAMELIS	haemorrhoids; varicose veins; bruising; tissue damage	swelling; engorgement
HEPAR SULPHURUS (HEPAR SULPH.)	coughs; croup; sore throats; tonsillitis; earache; bronchitis; boils; abscesses	irritability; hypersensitivity
HYPERICUM	bruises; nerve injuries (crushed fingers, coccyx, puncture wounds); post-operative pain	excessive pain
IGNATIA	emotional upsets and shocks; grief; hysteria; despair	erratic

REMEDY	USE FOR	KEYNOTES
IPECACUANA	nausea and vomiting; asthma; whooping cough; coughs; headaches	nausea with all symptoms
LEDUM	puncture wounds; animal bites; stings; black eyes	wounds discoloured and cold
LYCOPODIUM	indigestion; heartburn; flatulence and constipation; sore throats	symptoms worse on right side; lack of confidence
MAGNESIA PHOSPHORICA . (MAG. PHOS.)	colic; cramps; period pains; neuralgia; sciatica	spasmodic, darting pains; better with warmth
MERCURIUS	infections; tonsillitis; earache; toothache; mouth ulcers	offensive secretions; metallic taste in mouth
NAT. MUR.	colds; herpes; grief	weakness; fatigue; irritability
NATRUM SULPHURICUM . (NAT. SULPH.)	asthma; rheumatism; head injuries; warts; morning sickness; digestive problems	thick yellow catarrh; better in dry weather
PETROLEUM	psoriasis; skin eruptions	deep, painful cracks; yellow discharge
PHOSPHORUS	bleeding nose/gums; nausea or vomiting; diarrhoea; respiratory problems; painful larynx	bleeds and bruises easily
RHUS TOXICODENDRON . (RHUS. TOX.)	shingles; chickenpox; urticaria; mumps; sprains and strains; lumbago; sciatica; rheumatism	extreme restlessness; worse after rest; better after motion
RUTA	all strains and sprains; bruised bones; fractures; dislocations	lassitude
SABADILLA	hayfever	violent, spasmodic sneezing
SEPIA	menstrual complaints; menopause; morning sickness abscesses; wounds; splinters	debility; emotional indifference
SILICA	toothache; earache; headache; sinusitis; styes	slow healing; low vitality
STAPHYSAGRIA	cystitis; styes; eye infections; eczema; grief	resentment; suppressed anger; worse with touch
SULPHUR	skin conditions such as eczema, psoriasis, acne, boils	burning and redness; itchiness; worse with warmth of bed; worse after washing; self-centred
SYMPHYTUM	bone fractures; eye injuries	pricking pain
THUJA	infections; warts; styes; ill-effects of vaccination	exhaustion
URTICA URENS	urticaria; burns; scalds; chicken-pox; neuritis	burning; itching

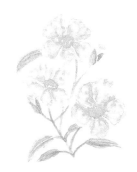

BACH FLOWER REMEDIES

The Bach flower remedies are made from the flowers of wild plants, bushes and trees of the British countryside. They are prescribed on the basis of mental rather than physical symptoms. It was the belief of Edward Bach, a medical doctor and homeopath, that negative emotions brought about physical disease (a fact recently acknowledged by medical science).

He therefore felt that mental symptoms rather than physical ones presented a more accurate indication of the cause of a disease, and should be used as the only guide to the correct treatment. He discovered 38 remedies which could successfully treat the gamut of negative emotions, from anxiety to apathy. Since then, new flower and tree essences have been developed around the world. The Flower Essence Society in California was established to research and provide information about these newly developed essences.

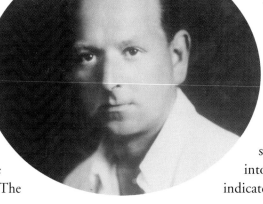

Above: *Dr Edward Bach (1880–1936) rediscovered the ancient art of using flower essences to heal negative emotional states. Bach used his well-developed intuitive abilities to select his comprehensive range of flower remedies.*

HOW TO SELECT THE RIGHT REMEDIES

Dr Bach intended his remedies to be used by everyone. They are totally without side effects and can be given to babies, the elderly, sick people on medication and animals. In treating yourself, try to honestly examine your predominant emotional traits and habits before selecting the remedies most suited to your temperament and current emotional problems. It is important that the combination includes your 'type' remedy – the one that most closely reflects your nature and personality. This can usually be gauged from your reactions under stresses such as severe fatigue or emergencies. For example, if stressful situations plunge you into feelings of self pity, Chicory is indicated as the 'type' remedy, whereas if you feel compelled to consult everyone's opinion before acting, Cerato, the remedy for self-doubt, is suitable. Often more than one 'type' remedy seems clearly indicated, as well as one or two others for specific problems which may be of a temporary nature (such as White chestnut for a preoccupation with a particular issue). It is recommended that no more than five remedies be combined at one time.

All the following remedy descriptions have their positive counterparts. For instance, the positive aspect of the self-centred 'Heather' type is an ability to put one's own troubles aside and to help others. The Bach flower remedies, by treating negative aspects which have developed because of stress and tension, allow the positive characteristics to unfold and dominate.

SELECTING FOR CHILDREN AND BABIES

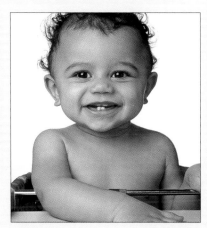

Babies' behaviours reflect their feelings. 'Chicory' babies are only truly pacified when they are being nursed; 'Clematis' babies live in a world of their own, often sleeping a lot; and 'Agrimony' babies only cry when something is wrong. Young children often battle through childhood with strong feelings of worry, resentment and jealousy. Their reaction to disease often reveals their type. The 'Water Violet' child will want to be left alone, while the 'Impatiens' child will be irritable and impatient. Bach felt it was important to treat these negative emotional aspects as soon as possible so that the child's positive nature could prevail.

TREATMENT INSTRUCTIONS

Bach flower remedies are widely available in a concentrated form known as a stock remedy. These should be stored in a cool, dark place and will last indefinitely. Individual mixtures are made from these stock remedies by adding 2 drops of each chosen remedy to a 20–30 ml (¾–1 fl oz) dropper bottle containing two-thirds water and one-third brandy (as a preservative). Mix well. Take a couple of drops of this mixture either in water (or in juice or food) or directly onto the tongue (don't touch the tongue with the dropper) four times a day. Improvement should be experienced, especially in mood and attitude, within two weeks. Continue with this mixture until you feel well, otherwise change the combination of remedies, especially if the emotional state alters during the course of treatment.

Below: *Dr Bach made his remedies by floating freshly picked flowers on spring water and exposing them to the sunlight for several hours. This charged the water with the flower's vibrational imprint – this subtle energy, by balancing the emotions, has a healing effect within the physical body.*

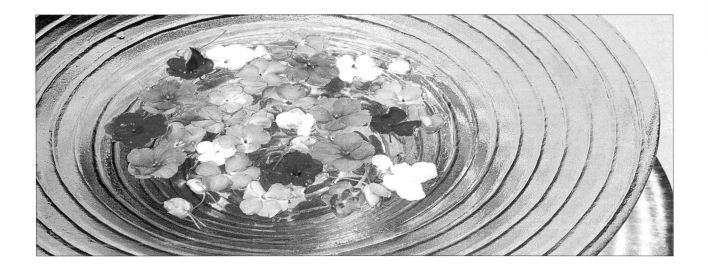

REMEDY DESCRIPTIONS

AGRIMONY . . . . .for peace-loving people who are distressed by quarrels and hide their worries and torments under a happy, carefree mask

ASPEN . . . . .for unaccountable fear, apprehension or anxiety, which is all the more disturbing for having no focus

BEECH . . . . .for intolerant people who are highly critical of others and quick to judge

CENTAURY . . . . .for kind, gentle people who are over-anxious to serve and please others. They are often exploited or imposed upon.

CERATO . . . . .for those people who doubt their own judgement, preferring constantly to seek the advice of others. They are often misguided as a result.

CHERRY PLUM . . . . . . .for over-strained people, near to a nervous breakdown, who fear they are losing their minds and might do something terrible

CHESTNUT BUD . . . . .for people who don't appear to benefit from experience or observation, making the same mistakes over and over again

CHICORY . . . . for possessive, over-protective and interfering people who always want their loved ones near them. They have a tendency to be self-centred and feel they are not appreciated enough.

CLEMATIS . . . . .for the daydreamers and the absent-minded who seem to pay little attention to their present circumstances and make little effort to get well

CRAB APPLE . . . . .for people who feel despair and disgust over their physical condition or some aspect of their nature. It is known as the cleansing remedy and is good for skin problems.

ELM . . . . .for capable people who become overwhelmed by their responsibilities and succumb to feelings of inadequacy

GENTIAN . . . . .for people who are easily depressed and discouraged by setbacks during an illness or in their daily affairs

GORSE . . . . .for those people who have totally lost heart and feel only great hopelessness and despair regarding their condition in life

HEATHER . . . . .for talkative, self-centred people who constantly seek companionship so that their grievances can be aired. They sap the vitality of those around them.

HOLLY . . . .(the 'Pandora's Box' remedy) for people who suffer from feelings of jealousy, envy, revenge, suspicion and hatred

HONEYSUCKLE . . . . . .for people who continually dwell in the past, feeling the present or future will never live up to the past. This is the remedy for homesickness.

HORNBEAM . . . . .for the type of mental fatigue and weariness which makes it hard to get out of bed in the morning and face the day

IMPATIENS . . . . .for quick, active, nervous people who become impatient and irritable at the slightest delay or hindrance

LARCH . . . . .for people who seldom attempt anything, believing they are always doomed to failure. They suffer from a total lack of confidence.

MIMULUS . . . . .for shy, timid people who suffer from such known fears as being alone, accidents, illness, death, and so on

MUSTARD . . . . .for people who are prone to black periods of depression, which descend without warning and for no apparent reason

OAK . . . . .for courageous people who never stop trying nor give up hope, even though they may despair of the outcome

OLIVE . . . . .for people who are totally exhausted and drained of all vitality by a long-standing illness or other serious problems

PINE . . . . .for people who are always apologizing and blaming themselves. They are never content with their achievements and feel guilty for not doing better.

RED CHESTNUT . . . . .for people who are overly anxious about others, frequently anticipating all sorts of mishaps and fearing the worst

ROCK ROSE . . . . .for anyone suffering extreme terror, fright or panic

ROCK WATER . . . . . . .for people who are rigid in mind, inflexible in opinion and self-denying in action. They are hard masters on themselves.

SCLERANTHUS . . . . . .for people who find it difficult to make a decision when there are two options. They suffer their indecision quietly, unlike the Cerato type. They tend to lack concentration and suffer from mood swings.

STAR OF BETHLEHEM for situations involving mental and physical shock: accidents, abuse of any kind, bad news and frights, serious disappointments, and so on

SWEET CHESTNUT . . .for people who suffer deep despair and loneliness. They are usually strong characters who bear their anguish quietly.

VERVAIN . . . . .for highly strung, active people who have strong opinions and ideas which they constantly try to impose on others. They are perfectionists and fanatics.

VINE . . . . .for people who are dominating, efficient and ambitious. They crave power and authority and expect obedience from all around them. They can be hard and cruel.

WALNUT . . . . .to help people through the various stages of life: teething, puberty and menopause. It is also for people who need to make a change (divorce, new job, new country, etcetera) but feel bound by old responsibilities and ties. (It is known as the link-breaker.) It is useful in helping to overcome addictions.

WATER VIOLET . . . . . .for people who in health and illness like to be left alone. These are usually quiet, gentle people who are self reliant and very capable. They often come across as being superior, proud or aloof.

WHITE CHESTNUT . . .for those who are tortured by persistent unwanted thoughts, often because of a preoccupation with a particular problem or event

WILD OAT . . . . .for talented and ambitious people who have become despondent and dissatisfied because they can't find an occupation which fulfills them

WILD ROSE . . . . .for people who are resigned to whatever happens and make little effort to change things for the better. They show no interest in life and make dull companions.

WILLOW . . . . .for people made bitter and resentful by their misfortunes. They begrudge other people's good fortune and feel life has been unjust to them. They seldom blame themselves.

RESCUE REMEDY . . . .a mixture of five of the flower remedies – Star of Bethlehem, Rock rose, Impatiens, Cherry plum and Clematis – was put together by Dr Bach for use in all emergency situations involving emotional shock, grief or acute stress of any kind.

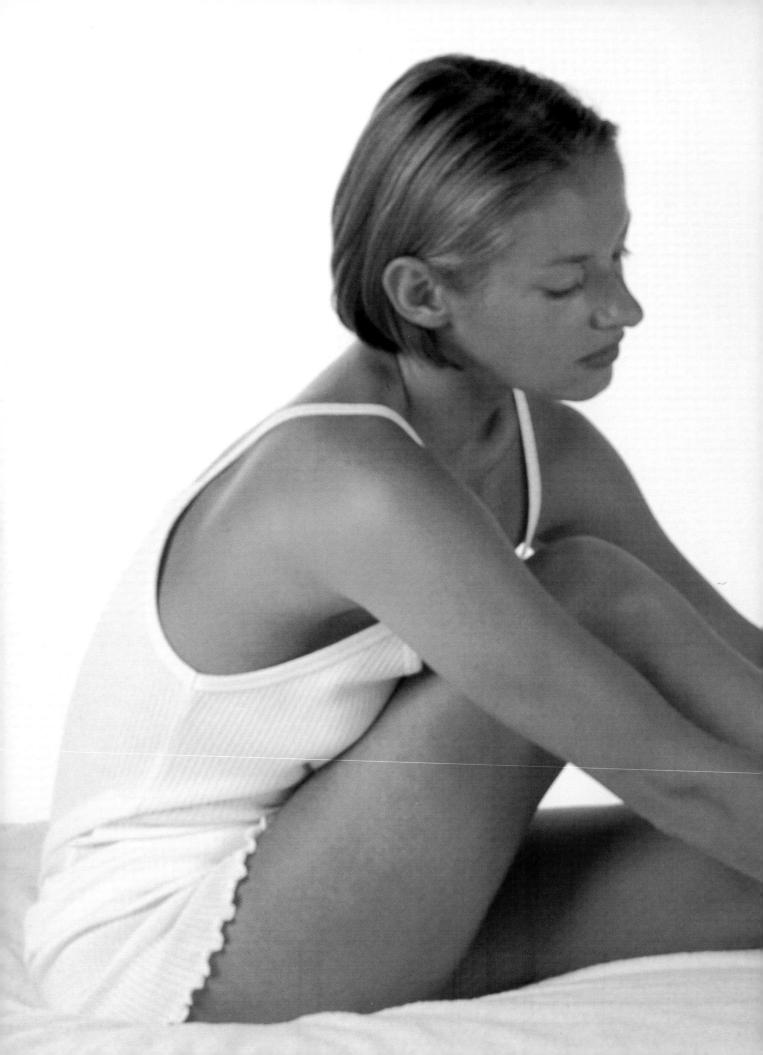

MANUAL THERAPIES

*H*ands can be used to communicate, comfort and to heal on many different levels. Touching, done with love and healing intent, induces profound relaxation as well as improvements in mood and self-esteem. It also reduces the levels of stress hormones in the body and enhances immune system activity.

Even a simple pat or hug can achieve similar healing responses which persist long after the physical action. This chapter explores how you can use the art of massage, a formalised system of touching, to heal yourself as well as other people. The wonderful benefits of massage can be further enhanced by using the acupressure techniques shown here. Acupressure, an ancient practice which originated in the East, involves applying deep finger pressure to specific points on the body to soothe and heal.

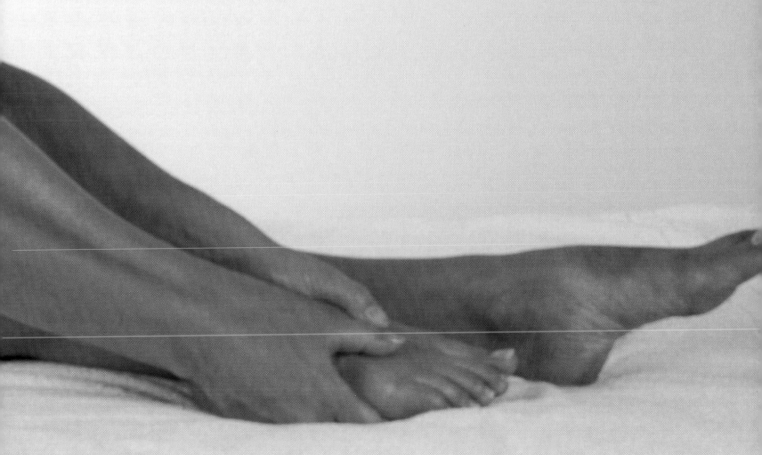

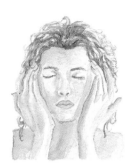

ACUPRESSURE

A cupressure is an ancient healing art using finger pressure on specific points of the body for disease treatment and prevention. It was widely practised over 3 000 years ago, first in China and then in Japan, where it is still used as a first-line treatment for pain and ill health. Many of us instinctively apply deep finger pressure to the top of our head, temples or the back of our neck when we have a headache, or to the area around our coccyx when we experience low back pain. This is a form of acupressure which, with a bit more knowledge and instruction, can become a very effective practice to add to the home store of natural remedies.

MERIDIAN NAMES

Lv	Liver	St	Stomach
TW	Triple Warmer	K	Kidney
H	Heart	LI	Large Intestine
GB	Gall Bladder	P	Pericardium
Sp	Spleen	B	Bladder
SI	Small Intestine	CV	Conception Vessel
Lu	Lung	GV	Governor Vessel

conception vessel

lung

stomach

spleen

Above: *These four meridian lines show how the invisible energy channels flow through the body.*

HOW ACUPRESSURE WORKS

The Chinese perspective

Centuries ago, Chinese healers noticed that if deep finger pressure was applied to painful or tender areas, other parts of the body also benefited. They found that various 'pressure points' affected the same area of the body as well as the functioning of a particular organ. These related pressure points are connected along energy channels called meridians, which are named after the associated organ. Fourteen different meridians, twelve of which run on both sides of the body, have been mapped out. These meridians course through the body, allowing the flow of Chi, the vital life-force. Disease and pain are thought to be the result of either blocked meridians or the unregulated flow of Chi. The practice of acupressure (and acupuncture) restores the proper flow of energy through the meridians, thereby restoring health and wellbeing.

The Western perspective

Western doctors have long known that massage or heat treatment on very tender points of the body can bring relief to painful conditions experienced elsewhere in the body. Over 70% of these 'trigger' points appear to coincide with acupressure (and acupuncture) points. Based on research findings which showed that it was possible to stop a pain signal reaching the brain, it was proposed that this is what happens when trigger points are stimulated. The 'gate theory of pain' states that the stimulation of one group of nerve fibres can close the gate on pain signals travelling along another group of fibres. It has also been discovered that the stimulation of these trigger points leads to the production of endorphins in the brain. Endorphins are the body's natural pain killers and may account for the long-term benefits of acupressure.

Trials have demonstrated the effectiveness of acupressure in the relief of a wide variety of ailments, including painful conditions, all types of nausea and asthma.

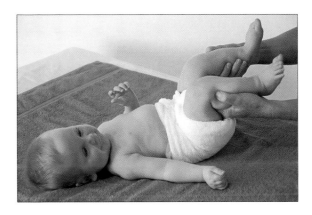

Above: *Acupressure is an effective home therapy, suitable even for babies. Here the Three Mile (St 36) point, located on the outside of the shin bone, is stimulated to relieve colic and boost immunity. As it is hard to locate exact points on babies, firmly rub around the entire area with the tips of your thumbs.*

ACUPRESSURE IN THE HOME

Acupressure is safe to do at home for a range of common complaints, but if the ailment persists then medical advice must be sought. You might occasionally experience a temporary worsening of your symptoms. This will not last and should lead to an improvement. The first stage of treatment is to make sure that you and the person you are treating are calm and relaxed. Any position which is comfortable can be adopted; clothing should be loose and fingernails trimmed.

Find the acupressure points recommended for the condition you wish to treat by following the instructions and diagram guidance in the self-treatment section overleaf. Most pressure points lie on a major band of muscle or in a hollow next to a bone. Don't worry about not being able to find the right point – gently prod around until you find the most tender spot in the area indicated.

Once you have located the point, slowly begin applying pressure with your thumb or middle finger pad, keeping your thumb or finger as upright as is comfortable. Keep increasing the pressure until it causes a pleasurable discomfort – but not pain. Different areas of the body will require different amounts of pressure. Hold a steady pressure for 1–2 minutes. The discomfort will often fade away after a minute or so. Finish off with a light, soothing touch. If you find it difficult to sustain finger pressure, use your fingertips, knuckles or even the heels of your hands to briskly and firmly rub the area.

Acupressure points can either be referred to by their meridian name and number, such as Liver 3 or Stomach 36 (pp. 70, 72–73), or by their much more inspiring Chinese names. For instance, Bigger Rushing relieves congestion and helps clear the system of toxins, while the Three Mile Point is famous for relieving fatigue and allowing people to go those extra miles! It is useful while pressing a point to take slow, deep breaths and to visualize the healing benefits of that point.

SHIATSU

Shiatsu, literally meaning finger pressure, is based on the same principles as acupressure and acupuncture. Although their origins are the same, shiatsu took on a form of its own over the many centuries it was practised in Japan. Today the treatment uses other massage and manipulative techniques as well as finger pressure.

POTENT PRESSURE POINTS TO REMEMBER

There are certain points which have a very powerful healing and rejuvenating effect on the mind and body, and these should become part of a regular routine to promote health and wellbeing. They are:

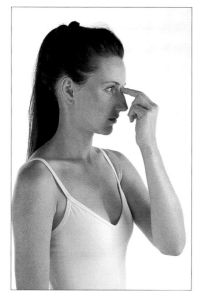

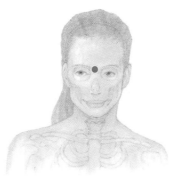

Third Eye (GV 24.5). This is a calming point that balances glandular function and relieves anxiety, irritability and depression. It is located between the eyes where the nose ends and the forehead begins.

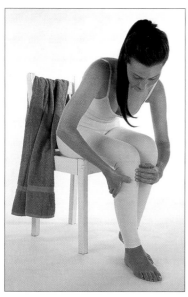

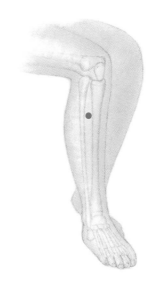

Three Mile (St 36). This point relieves fatigue, improves digestion and strengthens the immune system. It is located four fingerwidths below the kneecap and one fingerwidth to the outside of the shin bone.

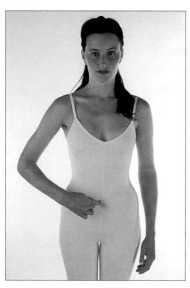

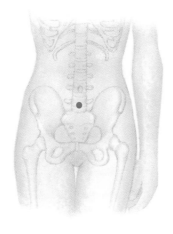

Sea of Energy (CV 6). This point revitalizes the body and strengthens the lower back. It is located three fingerwidths below the navel.

HOW TO STIMULATE ACUPRESSURE POINTS

For acute conditions press the recommended points several times an hour for a minute or more. Long-standing conditions will require up to 20 treatments. It is best to treat at least twice a day for the quickest results. Continue using the points on a regular basis (2–3 times a week) even when the condition has improved.

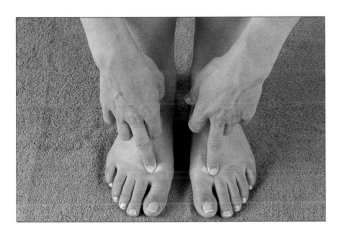

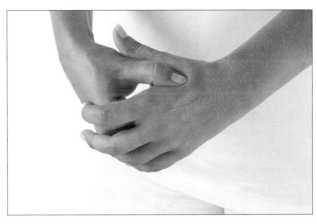

Bigger Rushing (Lv 3). This point relieves congestive and painful conditions. It is located in the valley between the big toe and the second toe.

Joining the Valley (LI 4). This point is useful for constipation and for reducing the pain of headaches, toothache and menstrual cramps. It is located in the webbing between the thumb and the fore-finger on each hand.

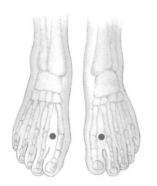

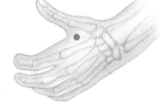

CAUTION

Acupressure is a safe, natural treatment for a wide variety of complaints, with the following provisos:

• Pressure points, especially if they are exceptionally tender, should be stimulated briefly (less than 30 seconds) and gently on anyone with a serious illness and during pregnancy.

• Joining the Valley (LI 4) should be avoided during pregnancy.

• Points which lie on inflamed or infected skin should be avoided.

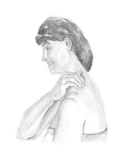

MASSAGE

The instinct to use hands to soothe, comfort and heal is so strong that the practice of massage must be as old as humankind. Formalized systems of massage were practised in China 5 000 years ago. In the West the healing art of massage never really flourished because of religious doctrines equating such activity with sin. The first formalized system was developed in Sweden by Per Henrik Ling during the early nineteenth century. By the middle of the century, massage, in combination with hydrotherapy, was part of the European health care system. It took another hundred years for Britain and America to realize the health benefits of massage. Massage is now widely available and is mostly based on or derived from the original Swedish massage techniques. It is simple to practise on yourself or others and should become a central part of your family life, as regular massages enhance both physical and mental health and relationships.

Dolores Krieger, professor of nursing at New York hospital, became fascinated with the idea that everyone could be taught to heal using touch. Work with well-known healers had demonstrated clear and measurable changes, such as an increase in haemoglobin levels after a healing session. She demonstrated that anyone could be taught to heal with touch; all that is required is a strong desire to help, practice and a good state of health. Her 'therapeutic touch' methods have been taught to thousands of caregivers throughout the world.

HOW MASSAGE WORKS

Touch is the fundamental medium of massage therapy. Any kind of touching, such as stroking, patting, squeezing and hugging, as well as specific massage techniques are associated with a multiplicity of benefits which are not all fully understood. However, research suggests that touch appears to be as essential to human growth and wellbeing as diet and exercise. Premature babies in incubators who are regularly massaged by their mothers show greater weight gain and nerve and brain development than babies who are not massaged. Adolescents who report lots of touching in their families are less inclined to be depressed, delinquent or aggressive. They also have greater self-esteem and a positive attitude to their bodies. Children who receive a daily massage show a much better immune response, have reduced levels of stress hormones, sleep better and are more cooperative.

BENEFITS OF MASSAGE

◆ Owing to the body's 'relaxation response' to massage, it reduces the effects of stress on the nervous system. Long-term stress can lead to a number of psychological symptoms (p. 87) such as anxiety, nervousness, depression and apathy. Massage can therefore achieve apparently contradictory effects – it will calm and soothe an anxious person but stimulate and energize a depressed one.

◆ It reduces muscle tension and spasm and may also lead to better postural habits.

◆ Massage increases circulation of blood and lymph. The increased blood flow brings more nutrients and oxygen to the area, while the improved movement of lymph ensures that excess fluid, cellular waste and foreign particles such as bacteria are eliminated.

◆ Massage increases the recovery rate of sore and aching muscles after vigorous exercise. (Lactic acid build-up in the muscles after strenuous exertion or exercise is responsible for muscle pain; massage speeds up its elimination.)

◆ It restores strength and mobility after injury and surgery, and helps to break down scar tissue and adhesions.

◆ Massage helps immobilized people to maintain muscle tone and blood circulation.

◆ Strong friction or pressure massage stimulates the production of endorphins, the body's natural pain killers, thus reducing acute and chronic pain.

◆ As massage improves blood supply, it improves skin tone.

METHOD

While there are a few situations where massage is inadvisable (refer to the cautionary notes), almost everyone will benefit from massage. There are no hard-and-fast rules, but the various strokes should be rhythmical and free flowing. It is best to begin and end with the slow, stroking movements. Experiment with the techniques which bring the greatest relief and pleasure to the recipient. Choose a warm room and make sure that both you and the person to be massaged are comfortable and relaxed. Use a lubricant such as sunflower or sweet almond oil and add one or two drops of the appropriate essential oils (pp. 47–49) to enhance the therapeutic effect. Warm the oil in your hands before applying it to the skin.

Effleurage (stroking)

With your fingers together and your thumbs outstretched, glide your hands slowly along the contours of the body in the directions illustrated on the right. Exert more pressure on the upward strokes and use soft fingertip pressure on the downward strokes. Repeat each movement several times. This technique reinforces the return flow of the blood to the heart and the movement of lymph.

CAUTION

Do not massage for the following conditions:
- serious heart disease
- phlebitis (inflammation of a vein)
- varicose veins
- fevers
- acute inflammatory conditions
- open, infected or bruised skin
- fractures
- osteoporosis

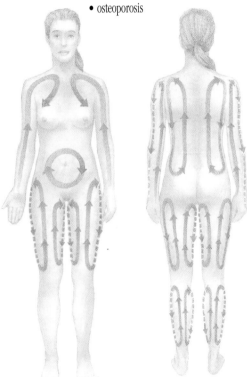

Above and below: *For effleurage, ensure that you massage in the direction of the arrows, using more pressure on the upward strokes and less on the downward strokes.*

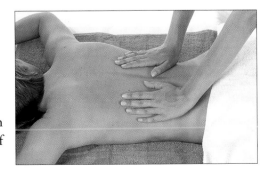

Kneading (petrissage)

Use the heels of your hands to apply firm downward pressure, then use the fingers and thumbs to squeeze and roll the soft tissue. Keep your hands close together, alternating them in a rhythmic fashion much as you would when kneading bread. Start from the midline and work outward, as illustrated. This technique stretches and relaxes tense muscles.

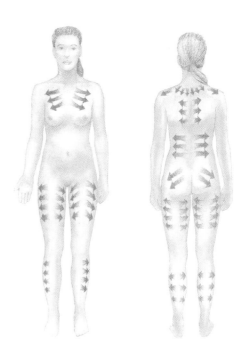

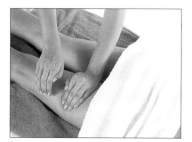

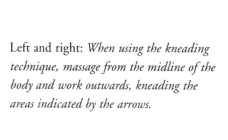

Left and right: *When using the kneading technique, massage from the midline of the body and work outwards, kneading the areas indicated by the arrows.*

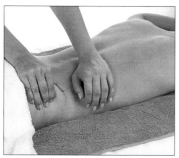

Kneading

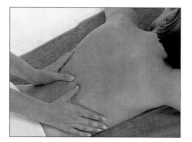

Percussion

Percussion

This involves the use of bouncy chopping or cupping strokes and can be very stimulating. Only use these strokes on the buttocks, thighs and calves and never on bony areas. The wrists should be loose and flexible and the hands shouldn't be raised more than 10 cm (4 in) from the skin. Alternating hands rhythmically, briskly strike the skin with the side of the palms or cupped hands. Move up and down the band of muscle. Always follow with effleurage.

Friction

This deep-tissue stroke should be done carefully, always gauging the person's response. Use the pad of your index finger or thumb to apply firm pressure in small circular movements for 10–20 seconds. Make sure you rotate the muscle and do not just move on the skin. Some people prefer to apply static deep pressure similar to acupressure techniques (pp. 70–73). Friction works well for shoulder muscles and for the muscles on either side of the spine.

Friction

Knuckling

Curl your hands into loose fists and then with the middle part of your fingers make small circular movements to create a continuous rippling effect. This movement is ideal for massaging feet, hands and shoulders.

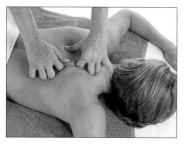

Knuckling

MASSAGE IN THE HOME

A full-body massage is indeed a therapeutic treat but is not always possible. If time is short, concentrate instead on the back and shoulder muscles where tension is greatest. If a back massage is out of the question, there is a range of other useful massage techniques which can be applied to yourself or someone else any time and anywhere.

Head massage

Place your thumbs behind your ears and spread your fingers out on your scalp. Without shifting the position of your fingers, make circular movements (friction) for 20 seconds so that your scalp moves over your skull. Move your fingers to a different part of the scalp and repeat. For tension headaches, place your thumbs on your temples and your fingers along the midline of your forehead. Make slow circular movements as above for 60 seconds.

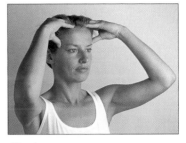

Head massage

Shoulder massage

Place your right hand on your left shoulder and squeeze and roll the shoulder muscle. Seek out tense, knotted areas and apply deep friction with your fingertips. Keep your chin tucked in, and make sure your shoulders are relaxed and not hunched up. Repeat with your left hand on your right shoulder.

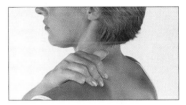

Shoulder massage

Finger and palm massage

Use your right thumb and index finger to squeeze and gently tug your left thumb. Start at the base and work your way around and up until you reach the very tip. Repeat for each finger and then change hands. Now interlace your fingers keeping your thumbs free. With your right thumb apply deep pressure to points all over your left palm, beginning at the base and moving up towards the fingers. Pay particular attention to the fleshy base of the thumb and the soft tissue between the finger bones. Repeat the process using your left thumb on your right palm.

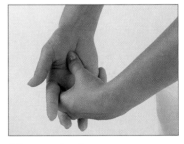

Finger and palm massage

Foot massage

Treating your whole body through a comprehensive foot massage is known as reflexology and is based on the premise that the feet (like other parts of the body) contain reflex zones linking them to the rest of the body. A simple foot massage has extensive thera-peutic benefits. First, warm the foot by rubbing it between your hands. Then massage each toe using the technique described for the finger massage. Hold your foot firmly and use the knuckling technique over your entire sole. Then use deep thumb pressure on every part of the sole, starting at the inside base and working straight up in a line towards your toes. Hold the pressure for half a second before sliding your thumb slightly forward to the next spot. Do not lift your thumb off the skin. When you reach the toes, begin again at the base just to the side of where you started. Repeat until you have covered the whole area.

REFLEX AREAS IN THE FOOT

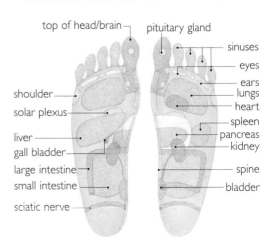

top of head/brain — pituitary gland — sinuses — eyes — ears — lungs — heart — spleen — pancreas — kidney — spine — bladder

shoulder — solar plexus — liver — gall bladder — large intestine — small intestine — sciatic nerve

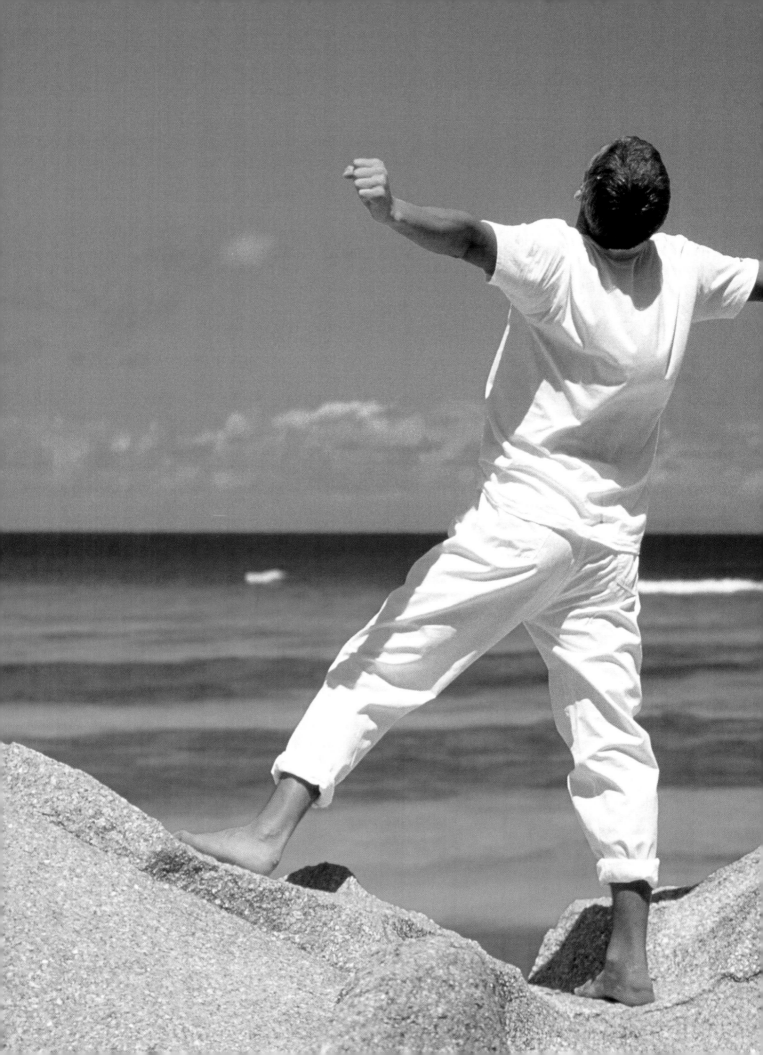

THE MIND AND HEALTH

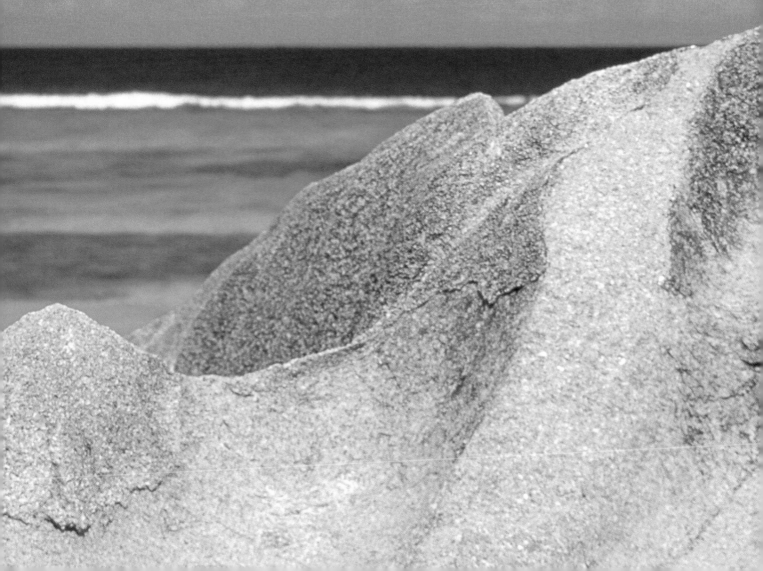

*T*he mind is the most powerful means we have by which to positively influence our health and general life experience. Everything we think and feel is determined by our basic attitude to life and how we react daily to people and events, particularly stressful events. Studies have shown that optimistic people see hope and beauty even in adversity, and maintain family and community relationships and a sense of useful purpose or faith. The immune system response is consistently stronger in optimists, who show less incidence of disease, improved recovery rates and reduced mortality when compared to pessimists. In fact, pessimists have been shown to feel more isolated and tend to see only that which reinforces their negative outlook. They react predominantly with feelings of hostility (even towards themselves), anxiety, hopelessness and depression. All of these feelings have widespread repercussions on biochemical processes. Fortunately, there are many ways of transforming our experience of life. Humour plays a vital role – laughter is a tremendous immune and mood enhancer; even forcing a smile has been shown to improve one's mood and emotional state. Becoming involved in communal or team activities and support groups are also significant ways to reduce feelings of isolation and to improve health and longevity.

This chapter explores several simple yet extremely effective techniques, ranging from meditation to relaxation and breathing exercises, which, in varying degrees, improve immune function, general health, response to stress, personal relationships and overall quality of life.

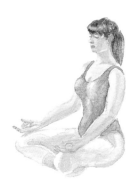

MEDITATION

Meditation is the act of achieving a state of consciousness in which the mind is totally still, yet alert. It is quite different to the more common definition of the word, which implies deep reflective thought on a subject. Many people, encouraged from an early age to keep their minds busy and occupied, find it difficult to enter this deliberate state of stillness. Over the centuries several techniques have been developed to help still the mind, and these have become part of the process of meditation. They are, however, only techniques, and should not be confused with the meditative state itself.

Meditation is neither a religious activity nor a form of hypnosis. It is a process of self-development that enhances mental and physical health, and is compatible with all doctrines, from secularism to Christianity.

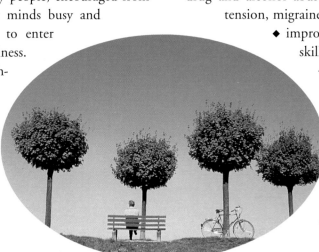

Above: *Meditation does not always have to take place indoors in the lotus postion! Once you become practised at it, any quiet spot outdoors where you will not be disturbed can provide an inspirational environment in which to relax, let go of stressful, circling thoughts and meditate. Practised regularly, it will confer profound mental and physical benefits.*

WHY MEDITATE?

Numerous scientific studies have demonstrated the benefits of meditation. Regular meditation is able to:

◆ reduce the effects of stress, and is therefore beneficial in stress-related disorders such as anxiety, depression, drug and alcohol abuse, insomnia, asthma, hypertension, migraine and skin problems;

◆ improve memory, problem-solving skills and creativity;

◆ increase energy levels;

◆ increase feelings of happiness and self-esteem;

◆ improve relationships;

◆ improve overall health;

◆ improve and speed up recovery from disease when used together with conventional treatment.

In short, the adoption of a regular routine of meditation is one of the single most important contributions you can make to your physical health and mental well-being and fulfillment.

WHAT HAPPENS DURING MEDITATION?

The 'relaxation response' is initiated during meditation, during which the following changes in the body occur:

- a significant decrease in heart rate;
- a reduction or stabilization of blood pressure;
- a slower, shallower breathing pattern;
- a dramatic reduction in muscle tension;
- a decrease in skin conductivity, reflecting a decrease in anxiety (anxiety increases skin conductivity, and this can be electrically detected – the operating principle behind lie detectors);
- changes in brain-wave activity, indicating an alert but relaxed state.

These beneficial effects are not confined to the period of meditation but continue throughout the day, effectively counteracting the negative biochemical results of stress build-up. Regular meditators have been shown to recover more quickly from stressful situations and to habituate faster to continuous stress (such as machinery or traffic noise) than non-meditating counterparts.

PROVEN BENEFITS

A study of 2 000 meditators matched with a control group found that, over a period of some five years, the meditating group were hospitalized for heart disease 87% less and for cancer 55% less than the control group.

HOW TO MEDITATE

- Set aside two periods of 10–20 minutes daily – one in the morning and one in the evening – avoiding times when you may be sleepy or have a full stomach. Set and muffle an alarm clock so that you do not have to worry about the time.
- Choose a quiet place where you'll be undisturbed. Try to establish a regular time and place – this makes meditation easier.
- Either sit on a straight-backed chair or on the floor in a cross-legged position. Make sure you are comfortably erect without straining any muscles. Rest your hands on your lap as shown (see right). If you are unable to sit, lie flat on your back in the 'corpse' position (p. 83).
- Close your eyes or keep them very slightly open if you struggle with drowsiness when your eyes are closed. Scan your body for any tension or tightness and release it. Breathe slowly and naturally through your nostrils.
- Choose one of the techniques on the following page (p. 82) for stilling the mind. Experiment freely before settling on the one which you find the most effective.
- On concluding your meditation, gently return your attention to your surroundings. Stretch out and relax. Note any effects the meditation has had but avoid judging it as good or bad: there is no right experience, just a personal one. Don't worry if nothing special seems to be happening. Use this period when the mind is quiet and receptive to visualize and make positive affirmations. Never come out of a meditation abruptly – your blood pressure drops during meditation and if you get up suddenly you may feel quite dizzy; you will also lose some of the benefits of meditation if you do.

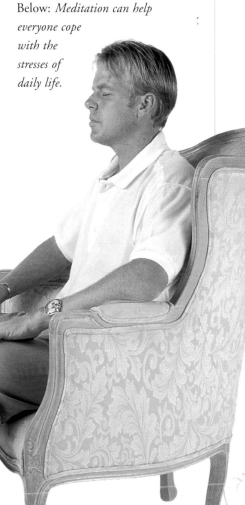

Below: *Meditation can help everyone cope with the stresses of daily life.*

MEDITATION TECHNIQUES

Focused breathing

Use your full attention to focus either on the rising and falling of your abdomen or on the air flowing in and out of your nostrils as you inhale and exhale. Let your breathing come naturally without any attempts to regulate it. As soon as you become aware that your attention has shifted to passing thoughts, images or emotions, gently return the focus to your breathing.

Breath counting

Breathing naturally, count each inhalation (or each exhalation), beginning at one and ending at ten. Repeat the process. If your mind wanders, simply begin counting from one again. This method gives your mind something to focus on and clearly indicates when your attention has wandered. It is a useful technique for people who find circling thoughts a problem.

Mantra or sound meditation

This method involves the silent repetition of a word or phrase to help still the mind. It can be a familiar, commonplace word (like 'one') or a word that holds significance (like 'peace'). Alternatively, you can use any words or phrases that are meaningful to you. Single words or short phrases are best. If you are comfortable with sacred and mystical sounds from other cultures, you can use the Sanskrit word 'om' (pronounced 'ome') – the supreme Hindu mantra. Another significant Sanskrit mantra is the sound 'hamsah' (meaning 'I am that'). As the incoming breath naturally makes the sound of 'ha' while the outgoing breath makes the sound of 'sah' (the 'm' occurring spontaneously at the transition), this is referred to as the 'natural' mantra. Simply become aware of this natural sound as you breathe in and out.

Once a mantra has been chosen, begin repeating it silently at a speed that feels comfortable. Match the rhythm of the mantra with your natural breathing pace.

Once your mind has become still, the repetition of the mantra becomes unnecessary. Observe any thoughts or images that come into your mind and then let them go. If your attention becomes caught up in your thoughts, start repeating the mantra again.

Concentrative meditation

Focus, without straining, on an object such as a lighted candle placed about 1 metre (3 feet) away at eye level. Try not to blink. Slowly close your eyes and visualize the object in your mind. When this 'after image' fades, open your eyes and start the process again. In the beginning you may find you spend much of your time with your eyes open. With time and practice it becomes easier to hold a mental image, and eventually the physical focal object can be dispensed with altogether.

POTENTIAL PROBLEMS

Some people report feeling anxious, physically uncomfortable, agitated or even nauseous. If this happens, open your eyes and relax, when you feel comfortable begin again. These experiences are usually confined to the first few attempts.

People may become discouraged because the meditation does not come up to their expectations, but there is no 'correct' experience. All that is required for success is regular practice. Most people in the West are unaccustomed to sitting in silence and it can come as a shock to discover how difficult it is to still the mind.

When the rational mind is stilled, thoughts and feelings – many of them negative and destructive – that have been buried in the subconscious may surface. These can be unpleasant, embarrassing or even shocking. Acknowledge them and then let them go by returning your focus to your breathing, mantra or object. Never try to suppress or drive them out, as this only serves to feed troublesome thoughts. Seek out the advice of an experienced teacher if you are concerned about anything you experience while meditating.

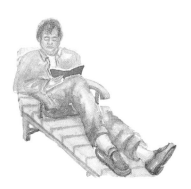

RELAXATION TECHNIQUES

Progressive muscle relaxation and breathing relaxation, techniques to be used upon awakening and before going to sleep, will help control the harmful psychological and physical effects of unresolved and prolonged stress. Both techniques elicit the 'relaxation response' (p. 81), reducing levels of stress hormones and muscle tension, stabilizing blood pressure and decreasing anxiety.

THE CORPSE POSITION
Lie on your back with your feet 40–50 cm (16–20 in) apart and your palms facing upwards roughly 20 cm (8 in) from your body. Let your legs and feet roll outwards. Check that your body feels balanced, then close your eyes and relax, focusing simply on the rise and fall of your abdomen.

PROGRESSIVE MUSCLE RELAXATION (PMR)

Find a quiet place to lie down – on the floor, on a mat or on a firm bed. Adopt the 'corpse' position and begin deep abdominal breathing (p. 83), sighing as you exhale. Feel the tension in your body release with each breath.

Now tense and relax each part of your body, beginning with your feet. Move

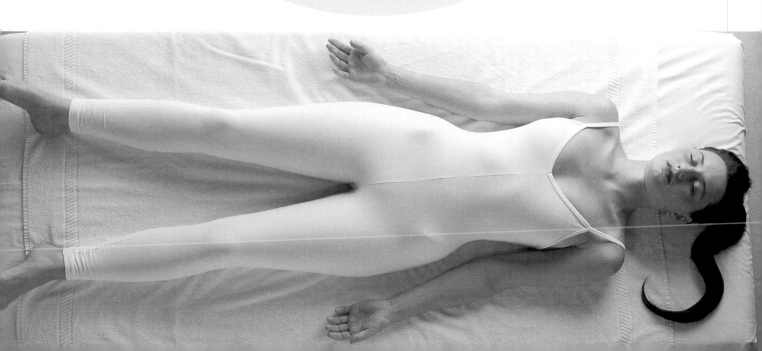

upwards through your legs, buttocks, stomach, back, shoulders, hands, arms, jaw and face. Tense each part as hard as you can for about 5 seconds, then relax for about 30 seconds, feeling the heaviness of that part as it comes to rest on the floor. Let your whole body go limp. Notice how different each area feels when tensed and then when relaxed. It may help to silently repeat the refrain 'my feet (or legs, buttocks, stomach, etcetera) are totally relaxed and feel heavy'.

Many people find this technique very effective for general body and mind relaxation, and use it for quick, spot-specific relief.

BREATHING RELAXATION

Most people take the act of breathing for granted and do not realize that the way they breathe can have widespread repercussions on their health. Breathing can be consciously controlled and used to treat stress-related ailments such as depression, fatigue, anxiety, insomnia, high blood pressure, gastrointestinal problems and asthma. The following technique should be practised several times a day and whenever you feel particularly stressed.

Standing, sitting or lying down, begin by vigorously exhaling through the nose. Then breathe in deeply through the nose, expanding (as fully as you can) first the abdomen, then the ribcage and finally the chest (this involves raising the shoulders). Do this to a comfortable count of eight. Exhale through the nose, also to the count of eight, first drawing in or contracting the abdomen, then the ribs and finally the upper chest (lowering the shoulders). Try to establish a flowing, wavelike pattern of expansion and contraction. Continue until you feel relaxed and calm.

When you become familiar with this pattern of breathing, hold your breath before exhaling to a count of eight. This enhances the widespread benefits of this breathing exercise.

Below: *For abdominal breathing, place one hand on your abdomen and the other on your upper chest. As you breathe, check that the hand on your chest remains motionless, while the hand on your abdomen is pushed upwards. It should only start to move once your abdomen is fully expanded.*

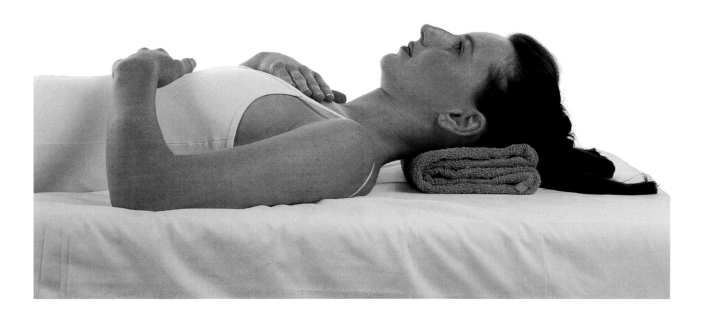

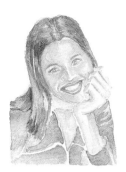

AUTO-SUGGESTION AND VISUALIZATION

Evidence of the role of mental attitudes and emotions in the development and progression of disease is so strong that all treatments should include a mental approach. The placebo effect (see below) is just one of the known ways in which positive suggestion can alter the course of disease. Auto-suggestion and visualization are simple but astoundingly effective techniques by which you can harness the healing powers of your mind and improve both your experience of life and your health.

THE PLACEBO EFFECT

The placebo effect describes the therapeutic benefits many people experience after a particular treatment due to the healing effect of believing the treatment will help rather than the treatment itself. Studies using placebos (pills/capsules with no pharmacologically active ingredients) to treat sick people show that 30 to 70% of those treated will experience relief – sometimes quite dramatic – of their symptoms. In addition it has been found that this healing response produces real and lasting benefits and is not just a temporary effect seen in gullible individuals (as many people allege). In fact, better-educated, more self-reliant people tend to show the best placebo response. Sadly, few efforts have been made to use or enhance this amazing healing response which is totally without side effects. All health practitioners, whether orthodox or complementary, owe a huge, largely unacknowledged, debt to the placebo effect. The time is long overdue for everyone to accept and use the power of the mind to positively influence health, through making use of readily available techniques such as visualization and auto-suggestion.

PRAYER AND FAITH

While this is a complex, emotive subject, from a health perspective there is no doubt that praying is good for you. During prayer the 'relaxation response' causes bio-chemical changes: heart rate and respiration slow down, blood pressure drops, muscle tension decreases and brain waves change. As with other techniques (such as meditation) which bring about this response, the benefits are not only physio-logical. According to one large study, the primary reported effect of prayer was a feeling of joy and awareness. Studies repeatedly show that people who draw comfort from religious faith have lower mortality rates – a fact which may, in part, be explained by the biochemical benefits of prayer.

AUTO-SUGGESTION

Auto-suggestion is a process of self-hypnosis whereby positive suggestions are implanted in the subconscious mind. A positive phrase (affirmation) is repeated 20 to 30 times several times a day. (The most famous phrase – suggested by Emile Coue, who is generally regarded as the 'father' of auto-suggestion – is 'every day, in every way, I am getting better and better'.) When repeated often enough, the conscious brain relegates this information to the subconscious, from where it will fundamentally influence your attitude, emotions and, ultimately, your physical health.

Any phrase can be used, but it should be constructed in positive terms (saying 'I am full of energy' is better than 'I am not tired'). You should repeat your chosen phrase last thing at night, first thing in the morning and whenever you remember to do so during the day. It must be repeated regularly to be effective. It is not unusual to feel foolish doing this, yet if you examine your thoughts closely you'll find that you do it naturally with a good many negative thoughts. Repeated phrases such as 'I'm not as good as . . .', 'I'm going to fail' and 'I can't cope' are commonplace and damaging refrains that influence every aspect of our lives. Turn all those phrases into positive ones – 'I feel good about myself', 'I'm going to succeed' and 'I am coping well' – and the rest will follow.

VISUALIZATION

Positive visualization as a therapy has ancient origins. However, although the ability is often highly developed in children, it is not encouraged, and many adults stop using their visual imaginations (except when they dream). Others use this facility in a destructive way, generating the emotions of fear and anxiety by always visualizing the worst outcome of any event (a journey ending in a car crash, an exam ending in failure, a disease ending in death, and so on). Imagining is such a powerful activity that the benefits can be similar to the actual experience. An experiment with a large number of people who had never before played basketball demonstrated this fact very well. After practising throwing the ball through the

Right: *To enhance your visualization skills, study this picture carefully for five minutes. Then close your eyes and try to recreate the picture in your mind's eye. Once you can do this easily, progress to imagining real-life scenes in which you are as you would like to be – healthy, happy, confident or in control.*

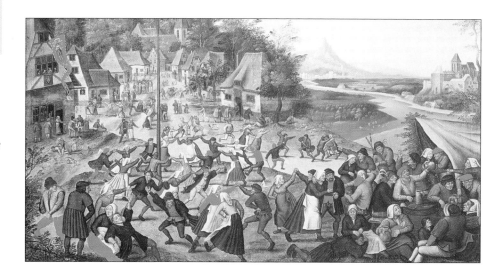

hoop for an afternoon, the group was divided into three. One group was not allowed to play any basketball, the second group was told to practise every day and the third group was told to visualize throwing the ball through the hoop every day. After one month the first group showed no improvement, but the second and third groups demonstrated an almost identical improvement in skill! This suggests that positive visualization can have far-reaching effects in every arena of your life: health, work, sport and social life. All you have to do is to visualize yourself as whatever you would like to be and you'll be that much closer to achieving your goals.

Many people struggle to visualize and need to be taught how to do so. One of the most effective ways is to look at a very detailed picture for five minutes, then to close your eyes and try to visualize each small part in turn. Open your eyes as soon as the image fades, look again and try to observe even greater detail which will help you visualize. As soon as you can successfully recreate a mental picture of the item, progress to imagining real-life scenes. (Some people seem unable to function in an imaginative visual mode but are nevertheless able to create effective 'imaginary' experiences using different sensory modes, such as hearing or feeling. These can be as effective.)

POSITIVE VISUALIZATION

◆ Before any event or activity, visualize yourself performing as well as you wish to.

◆ When you get sick, visualize yourself as well again. Don't dwell on how sick you feel and how you're missing out on things. Optimistic people have been shown to have a greater immune response than pessimists.

◆ Always think of your body as stronger than a disease you may be suffering from. The Simontons, cancer specialists, encouraged their patients to visualize a victorious battle going on between their more powerful immune cells and the invading but weaker cancer cells. Patients who used this method lived an average of a year longer than patients who did not visualize in this way. Use the images or symbols that work best for you.

STRESS – GOOD OR BAD?

Stress is a vital aspect of our survival and life experience, and can stimulate creativity and resourceful change; most people can relate periods of personal growth to some particularly stressful time or event. But for many of us stress remains unresolved, and this leads to the development of disease. Stress primes the body to cope with a challenging event, in what is often referred to as the 'fight or flight' response. Through the release of the so-called 'stress' hormones – adrenalin, noradrenalin and cortisol – the following changes occur which prepare the body for intense physical activity:

◆ breathing rate increases to take in more oxygen;

◆ heart rate and blood pressure increase in order to supply more blood to the muscles (for extra work) and to the brain (for quick, clear decision-making);

◆ the liver breaks down stored glycogen, releasing sugar for more energy;

◆ perspiration increases in order to keep the body cool;

◆ digestive processes stop.

These changes are good if they are followed by some appropriate physical activity (such as exercise). However, if the stress response is prolonged and unresolved (for example, if you are constantly frustrated at work and can do nothing about it), then both physical and mental health begin to deteriorate. People vary enormously in their ability to cope with stress, some even thriving on the resultant state of physical arousal. Many, however, do not. Warning symptoms of a stress overload may include any of the following emotional, behavioural and physical symptoms:

◆ depression, panic attacks, irritability, irrational outbursts, indecision and low self-esteem;

◆ increased deviant behaviour, smoking and drinking, nail- and lip-biting, grinding of teeth, and constant finger- or foot-tapping;

◆ high blood pressure, headaches, insomnia, diarrhoea and an increased susceptibility to infections and allergies.

Relaxation techniques, exercise and massage are some of the most effective ways of counteracting the harmful effects of unresolved stress. They are especially important in situations where it may be impossible to remove the source of stress, such as after the death of a loved one, during a very demanding or boring job or during prolonged periods of time spent looking after small children.

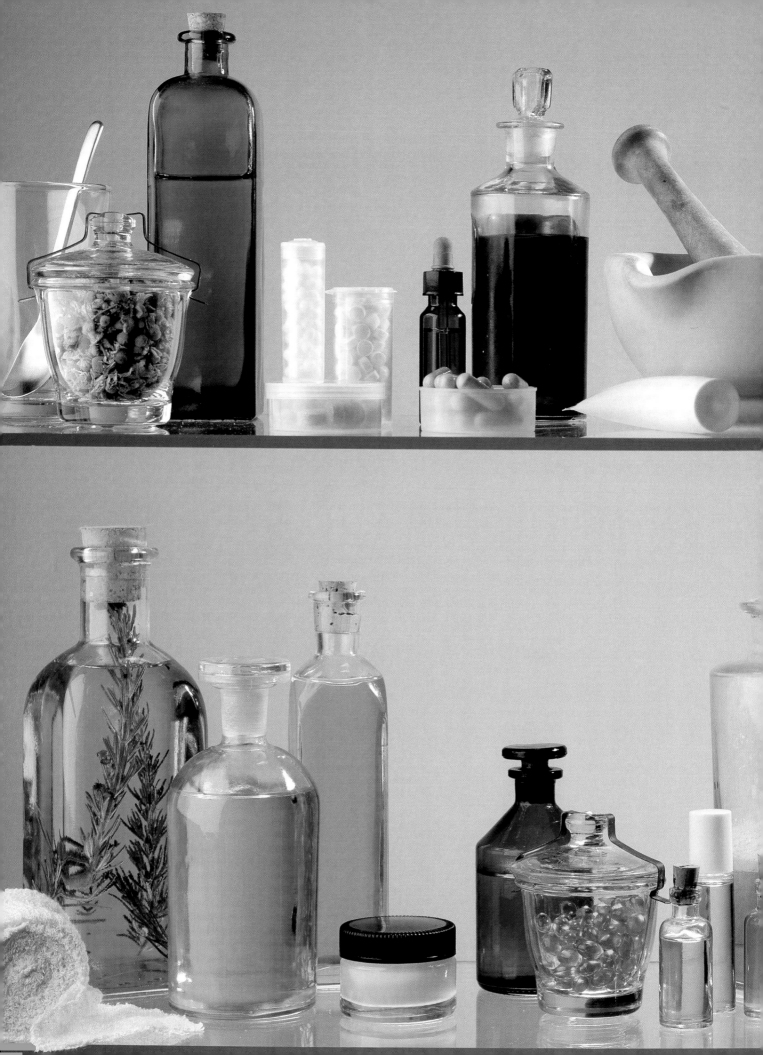

AILMENT AND TREATMENT GLOSSARY

*M*ost, if not all, complementary therapists would agree that a healthy diet, regular exercise and the practice of some form of relaxation are fundamental to maintaining a healthy mind and body, and we strongly recommend that everyone include all three as the basis of a healthy lifestyle. In recommending remedies for specific ailments in this section of the book, we have chosen to mention individual treatments where we feel they are essential to bring about relief. We mention the treatments which, in our experience, have produced the most reliable results. Please refer to the relevant chapters for further treatment indications. Unless stated otherwise, supplement dosages suggested are to be taken daily.

But just as disease and ill-health cannot be ascribed to one factor alone, so the treatment recommendations involve several different approaches. It is not necessary, however, to follow every directive. Depression, for example, could be cured simply by adopting a programme of regular exercise, or it might be alleviated by supplements of vitamins B and C, or a course of St John's wort. We suggest you experiment and find the combination that works best for you.

In addition, several herbal remedies are often recommended where perhaps one would suffice. This has been done to give you more freedom of choice, and to offer alternatives if a particular herb is unavailable in your area. All of the advice given needs to be followed for a minimum of six weeks before beneficial results for chronic complaints can be expected. If no improvement occurs within three months, we advise you to consult a professional.

GENERAL CAUTIONS

- Before embarking on any treatment, please read the chapter pertaining to that therapy, paying particular attention to the general cautions. Certain treatments carry very specific cautions and, where possible, page references have been provided to guide you; make sure that you read the relevant chapter and familiarize yourself with the necessary precautions.
- Only mild or stabilized conditions should be treated at home. Never stop any medications suddenly, but phase them out gradually with the help of your medical practitioner. With the exception of a few herbs and supplements where caution is specifically advised, all treatments described are compatible with orthodox treatment.
- Pregnant women should read the pages on pregnancy (pp. 96–97) first, before embarking on any course of treatment.

DOSAGE

- With the exception of the chapter dealing with childhood complaints, all supplement directions pertain to a daily ADULT dose. Do not exceed recommended dosages without professional advice. Children under 12 should take half the recommended dosage. Supplements for children under two years old should first be approved by a medical practitioner.
- It is impossible to recommend precise dosages for commercial herbal preparations, as they come in so many forms and strengths. Always follow the dosage directions supplied with any product. Dosages for home-made herbal preparations are supplied on p. 34 of the chapter on *Herbal Healing*.
- If no dosages are supplied in the relevant section of text, follow the manufacturer's instructions.

CHILDHOOD COMPLAINTS

The following advice is offered as a first line of treatment; if the child fails to respond within 24 hours and/or his or her condition suddenly deteriorates, consult a medical practitioner without delay.

CAUTION Use only pasteurized honey for children under one year old, as there is a very small risk that raw honey may contain bacterial botulism spores which could germinate in an immature intestine.

THE IMMUNE-SYSTEM-STIMULATING REGIME

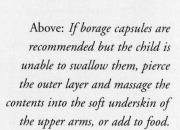

DIET
- Increase intake of fruit, vegetables, pulses and wholegrains.
- Reduce animal fat intake and restrict or eliminate all dairy products.
- Eliminate all sugar, processed foods and foods and drinks containing caffeine, colorants and flavourants.
- While the child is feverish, restrict the diet to fresh fruit (juiced if preferred), vegetables (raw or cooked in a soup) and filtered or mineral water.

SUPPLEMENTS
Multivitamin and mineral supplement
Vitamin C 200 mg twice daily. Chewable forms must be taken with food to avoid damage to dental enamel.
Zinc 1 mg per kg of body weight up to 10 mg

HERBAL
Echinacea (p. 39)
Garlic (p. 36)
Chamomile (p. 43)
Astragalus (p. 36)

NOTE: If a child is too young to swallow tablets, crush them between two spoons and mix the powder with some food or honey (see cautionary note, above).

Above: *If borage capsules are recommended but the child is unable to swallow them, pierce the outer layer and massage the contents into the soft underskin of the upper arms, or add to food.*

INFECTIONS

Most childhood infections are caused by viruses, against which antibiotics are useless. If a child suffers recurrent infections, his or her immune system is evidently compromised for one or more of the following reasons: nutritional deficiencies, a food or chemical allergy (especially if the child produces a lot of mucus) and stress. Check that he or she is not anxious about something or unhappy at school. If the stress is unavoidable, regular, non-competitive exercise, a soothing massage with lavender or chamomile oil and the appropriate flower remedies can work wonders. Otherwise the best approach is to boost the child's immune function: follow the immune-system-stimulating regime (above).

COLDS AND INFLUENZA (viral)
See p. 131.

MUMPS (viral)
GENERAL
Follow the immune-system-stimulating regime (above).
HOMEOPATHY
Aconite if symptoms appear suddenly and the child is anxious, restless and thirsty
Belladonna if the child is hot, flushed and has throbbing, swollen glands
Mercurius if the child is hot, sweaty and dribbling and has bad breath
Give 30C of chosen remedy four times daily.

CROUP (95% viral)
GENERAL
Follow the immune-system-stimulating regime (p. 90) if croup recurs frequently.
HOMEOPATHY
Aconite
Spongia or Hepar sulph. if Aconite does not work within 30 minutes
Give 30C of chosen remedy every 10 minutes until relief is obtained.
AROMATHERAPY
Eucalyptus oil. Massage 2 drops essential oil diluted with 2 tbsp carrier oil into the chest, or place 5 drops eucalyptus oil in a bowl of steaming water near the child to humidify the atmosphere.

EARACHE/OUTER EAR INFECTION
See p. 107.

MIDDLE EAR INFECTION
(30–50% bacterial)
GENERAL
Follow the immune-system-stimulating regime (p. 90) if ear infections are chronic, and exclude all dairy products from the child's diet.
HOMEOPATHY
Aconite if symptoms appear suddenly and the child is anxious, restless and thirsty
Belladonna if the child is hot and flushed and has throbbing, very painful ears
Chamomilla if the child is bad-tempered as a result of the pain and needs to be carried constantly
Pulsatilla if the child is weepy and clingy, with symptoms which keep changing
Give 30C of chosen remedy every 30 minutes until relief is obtained.

CHICKENPOX (viral)
GENERAL
Follow the immune-system-stimulating regime (see box on p. 90).
HOMEOPATHY
Rhus. tox. if very itchy, restless and distressed
Give 30C four times daily.
HERBAL
Calendula or echinacea. Apply lotion or cream to spots.

MEASLES (viral)
GENERAL
Follow the immune-system-stimulating regime (p. 90).
HOMEOPATHY
Aconite for sudden onset of fever with restlessness and anxiety
Ferrum phos. for early stages when symptoms are not yet pronounced
Gelsemium if the symptoms resemble flu, with aching muscles, shivering and drowsiness
Pulsatilla if the rash is followed by thick nasal discharge and crusty eyes and the child is weepy and clingy
Give 30C of chosen remedy four times daily.

WHOOPING COUGH (bacterial)
HERBAL
Echinacea
Liquorice (p. 40, caution)
HOMEOPATHY
Drosera
Bryonia if Drosera does not help within 30 minutes
Give 30C every 10 minutes until relief is obtained.

NAPPY RASH
See hyperactivity (p. 92) with regard to possibility of food or chemical allergy. Change nappies frequently, keeping the nappy off for as long as possible. Nappy rash may be due to a fungal infection or a contact irritation. Make sure nappies are well rinsed after washing and don't use fabric softeners or talcum powder.
HERBAL
Calendula (p. 39). Apply ointment frequently to affected area.
AROMATHERAPY
Tea tree oil. Massage 2 drops essential oil mixed with 2 tbsp olive oil into affected area.

TEETHING
HOMEOPATHY
Chamomilla if the baby is extremely irritable and bad-tempered but is helped by being carried
Pulsatilla if the baby whimpers or whines and is clingy
Give 30C of chosen remedy every 30 minutes until relief is obtained.

COLIC

Infantile colic is often due to an intolerance to cows' milk and is therefore more common in bottle-fed babies. However, breast-fed babies are not immune, as certain cows' milk proteins from the mother's diet can be present in the breast milk. If the baby also suffers from skin problems such as eczema and digestive and sleep disorders, the mother should try excluding dairy products from her diet. If that doesn't help she should rotate her consumption (and that of her baby's, if appropriate) of major foods, such as wheat (pp. 19–21), and keep a diary of her baby's colic attacks to identify any links. Allow up to 12 hours for a reaction to occur.

DIET
A soya milk substitute is recommended for bottle-fed babies, but obtain specialist advice first.

HERBAL
Fennel, chamomile, peppermint or rooibos. Give 3–4 tbsp herbal infusion every 2 hours, or 3 tbsp in a bottle three times daily before meals.

AROMATHERAPY
Chamomile oil. Gently massage abdomen in a clockwise direction with 2 drops essential oil in 2 tbsp carrier oil.

HOMEOPATHY
Chamomilla if the child is very irritable and angry
Dioscorea or Colocynthis if Chamomilla doesn't help
Give 30C every 10 minutes until the pain subsides.

SLEEPLESSNESS

See hyperactivity (right) with reference to possibility of food or chemical allergy.

SUPPLEMENTS
Give the supplements recommended for hyperactivity, ensuring that the multivitamin and mineral supplement contains 2 mg manganese.

HERBAL
Californian poppy
Chamomile

HYPERACTIVITY/ATTENTION DEFICIT DISORDER (ADD)

This is an umbrella term for a range of problems including one or more of the following: the child has a reduced concentration span, is demanding and easily frustrated, cries often and has frequent temper tantrums, is clumsy, is always touching things, is overactive and excitable, displays explosive and unpredictable behaviour or is restless, never wanting to sleep or waking up often.

Two-thirds of all cases of hyperactivity and childhood insomnia are caused by food and chemical allergies. If the child also suffers from headaches, skin problems (eczema, nappy rash, dry, patchy skin, cracked lips, dandruff or cradle cap), asthma, hayfever, bedwetting, aching legs, gastrointestinal problems (bloating, diarrhoea, constipation or colic), inappropriate fatigue, excessive sweating, cravings for sweet foods, a constantly runny nose and frequent infections, then a food or chemical allergy is the likely cause. Commonly implicated substances are cows' milk, food preservatives and colorants (also present in many medicines), wheat, chocolate, sugar, eggs and citrus fruits.

Try the following remedies. If they do not help, suspect a candida infection (see p. 130), particularly if the child was previously frequently treated with antibiotic medication.

DIET
Follow the basic guidelines for healthy eating (p. 13), taking care to exclude all junk food.

SUPPLEMENTS
Multivitamin and mineral supplement
Calcium 100 mg
Magnesium 100 mg
Zinc 1 mg per kg of body weight up to 10 mg
Vitamin C 200 mg twice daily
Borage oil (p. 17) 500 mg capsules twice daily

CRADLE CAP

See hyperactivity (above) for possibility of a food or chemical allergy.

AROMATHERAPY
Tea tree oil. Massage 2 drops essential oil mixed with 2 tbsp olive oil into scalp.

FEMALE COMPLAINTS

CYSTITIS

A condition characterized by painful, frequent passing of urine (which may be cloudy and smelly). There may also be pain in the lower abdomen, fever and general malaise. The infecting organism is usually spread from the anus, so good personal hygiene is important; wipe from front to back after going to the toilet. Don't use perfumed toiletries in this area and do wear cotton underwear. Frequent sexual intercourse can increase the chances of infection ('honeymoon' cystitis). Recurrent cystitis in which no infective organism is involved can be due to a food allegy (pp. 19–21) or candidiasis (p. 130). Serious cases may require a course of antibiotics.

DIET

Follow the guidelines for healthy eating (p. 13), taking care to avoid sugar (including all sweetened food and drinks) and caffeine. Reduce intake of animal fat. Eat plenty of fresh vegetables and fruit and drink plenty of water. Drink 1–2 glasses of pure cranberry juice daily as a preventative.

SUPPLEMENTS

Multivitamin and mineral supplement

Vitamin C 200 mg twice daily

Zinc 15 mg

HERBAL

Echinacea

Garlic

Buchu

Uva Ursi (p. 36, caution)

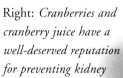

Right: *Cranberries and cranberry juice have a well-deserved reputation for preventing kidney stones and urinary tract infections. They not only acidify the urine, which discourages bacterial growth, but they also contain factors that envelop bacteria and prevent them from establishing a foothold in the urinary tract.*

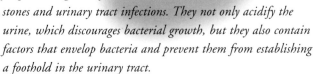

INFERTILITY AND MISCARRIAGES

These are complex issues which may be due to several factors, some of which cannot be helped. However there are several self-help measures that *may* address an underlying cause that is preventing conception or full-term carriage of the foetus. Deficiencies in vitamin E, zinc, manganese and fatty acids and an overload of toxic metals (p. 25) have been implicated in failure to conceive and miscarriages. Stress is a contributory factor and should be addressed with a programme of regular relaxation exercises, aerobic exercise and positive visualization.

DIET

Follow the guidelines for healthy eating (p. 13), taking care to exclude refined carbohydrates, sugar and margarine and cut down on animal fats. Alcohol, caffeine and tobacco should be excluded.

SUPPLEMENTS

Multivitamin and mineral supplement

Vitamin B complex

Vitamin C 200 mg twice daily

Vitamin E (p. 26, caution) 600 IU

Zinc 30 mg

Seaweed/algae supplement as directed (p. 25)

Flaxseed oil 1 tbsp

HERBAL

Dong quai (p. 36, caution)

Use as a female tonic to regulate the hormonal cycle.

AROMATHERAPY

Clary sage oil. Add 10 drops to 2 tbsp carrier oil and ask your partner to give you a relaxing full-body massage.

VAGINAL THRUSH

This is a disorder caused by an overgrowth of the Candida albicans yeast, resulting in vaginal irritation and a white discharge. It is particularly common after a long course of antibiotics. See advice for treating candidiasis (p. 130). Soak a tampon in live yoghurt and insert into the vagina; change four times daily.

AROMATHERAPY

Tea tree oil. Mix 20 drops essential oil with 3 tbsp tepid water and use as a douche, or apply mixture to a tampon, insert and change four times daily.

MENSTRUAL PROBLEMS

The menstrual cycle is dependent on a complex interplay of hormones and is quite easily upset by factors such as poor nutrition, illness and physical and psychological stress.

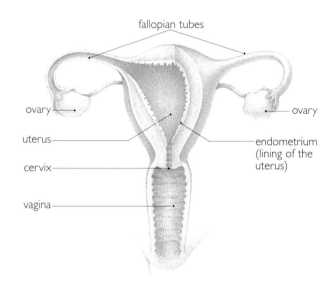

Above: *Female reproductive organs.*

CAUTION Any vaginal bleeding between periods or after menopause must be investigated immediately.

DYSMENORRHOEA (painful periods)
MENORRHAGIA (excessive blood loss)
SPOTTING AND IRREGULAR PERIODS

These are usually caused by hormonal imbalances or psychological stress.
DIET
Follow the guidelines for healthy eating (p. 13).
SUPPLEMENTS
Multivitamin and mineral supplement
Magnesium 200 mg
Flaxseed oil 1 tbsp or fish oil (p. 18, caution) 2 g
HERBAL
Dong quai (p. 36, caution) or agnus castus (p. 44, caution) to regulate periods
Cramp bark/raspberry for painful periods
RELAXATION
Some form of regular relaxation and exercise should be practised to reduce the possible contributory effects of stress.

AMENORRHOEA (loss of periods) AND SCANTY PERIODS

These conditions can result from slimming diets, excessive physical exercise or after coming off the contraceptive pill. Oestrogen levels are usually depressed and this adversely affects the deposition of calcium in the bones. Temporary amenorrhoea is not harmful, but in the long term it can increase vulnerability to osteoporosis. (Of course, amenorrhoea may also indicate pregnancy!)
GENERAL
Follow the advice given for dysmenorrhoea (see left).

PREMENSTRUAL SYNDROME (PMS)

This problem – also sometimes referred to as 'premenstrual tension' – affects up to 40% of women in their thirties and forties. It describes a range of symptoms which begin about a week before the period is due, and can vary from mild to severe. Symptoms include mood swings, irritability, depression, altered sex drive, headache, breast pain, backache, abdominal bloating and oedema of fingers and ankles. It is commonly due to an increased oestrogen-to-progesterone ratio.
DIET
It is important to reduce the intake of saturated fats (meat and dairy products) and salt and to eliminate sugar, refined foods, artificially saturated fats (margarine) and caffeine. The diet should be predominantly vegetarian and rich in fresh vegetables, fruit, wholegrains and pulses.
SUPPLEMENTS
Multivitamin and mineral supplement
Vitamin B$_6$ 50 mg
Vitamin E (p. 26, caution) 400 IU
Calcium 250 mg twice daily
Magnesium 200 mg twice daily
Zinc 15 mg
Flaxseed oil 1 tbsp or fish oil (p. 18, caution) 2 g
HERBAL
Agnus castus (p. 44, caution)
Dong quai (p. 36, caution)
Black cohosh (p. 39, caution)
Sage (p. 43, caution)
EXERCISE
Regular exercise has been shown to cause a dramatic reduction in PMS.

MENOPAUSE

Menopause, which signals the permanent cessation of the menstrual cycle, usually occurs between the ages of 45 and 50. There is a decrease in the level of oestrogen in the blood, which may lead to hot flushes, night sweats, vaginal dryness and atrophy, headaches, heart palpitations and osteoporosis. Associated pyschological symptoms include depression, lack of concentration and fatigue.

Few people realize that menopause is not a phase like puberty but a continued state for the rest of a woman's life. This is why herbal alternatives are superior to hormone replacement therapy, which is associated with serious health effects when used over many years. Women under 40 who have had hysterectomies with one or both ovaries still remaining may also experience menopausal symptoms due to insufficient oestrogen production.

DIET
Follow the guidelines for healthy eating (p. 13) and include lots of fresh fruit, vegetables and pulses.

SUPPLEMENTS
Multivitamin and mineral supplement
Vitamin C 200 mg twice daily
Vitamin E (p. 26, caution) 400 IU
Calcium 500 mg twice daily
Magnesium 300 mg twice daily
Zinc 15 mg
Flaxseed oil 1 tbsp

HERBAL
Black cohosh (p. 39, caution)
Agnus castus (p. 44, caution)
Dong quai (p. 36, caution)
Sage (p. 43, caution)

Left: *Soya beans, like the herbs agnus castus, dong quai, black cohosh and sage, are very rich in phytoestrogens. Phytoestrogens are plant compounds which balance the effects of oestrogen. They bind to and block oestrogen receptor sites in the body, thus reducing the negative effects of high levels of oestrogen (such as PMS and certain cancers). However, as they have a mild oestrogenic effect of their own, they can also help when oestrogen levels are low, such as in menopause and osteoporosis.*

OSTEOPOROSIS

After the age of 50 both men and women begin to lose calcium from their bones, making the bones more prone to fracture. The rate of loss is much greater in women owing to the effects of menopause (see left). Women should follow the supplement and herbal advice given for menopause. This regime will halt and even reverse the loss of bone mass. A regular exercise programme should also be adopted, as this increases bone density (p. 52). Men who suffer from osteoporosis should follow this advice, but exclude the herbal remedies that are recommended for women.

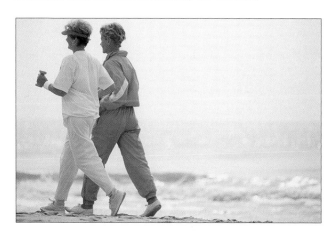

Above: *Walking helps to maintain strong bones and is safe, making it the best exercise for preventing osteoporosis.*

THE CONTRACEPTIVE PILL
The contraceptive pill usually consists of a combination of oestrogen and progesterone, and works by preventing ovulation. Although it is safer than it used to be, the pill still has an adverse effect on many nutrients and is associated with an increased incidence of cancer of the breast, cervix and liver. It also appears to increase the chances of a stroke or heart attack, high blood pressure, diabetes, gall bladder disease, food allergy, migraine, candidiasis and depression. Smoking and obesity increase the risk of these side-effects. If you are over the age of 45, still menstruating and taking the pill, it is important to be regularly monitored by a doctor. This is of particular importance if you have a family history of breast cancer.

PREGNANCY AND CHILDBIRTH

General advice and cautions are supplied for each therapy. For advice regarding problems such as constipation, indigestion and nausea, refer to the appropriate sections.

IMPORTANT: All remedies should first be agreed upon by your doctor.

DIET

Follow the basic guidelines for healthy eating (p. 13) and ensure an adequate intake of protein in the form of fresh fish or skinless poultry. If you are vegetarian, eat plenty of pulses and wholegrains. Coffee and tea consumption should be kept to a minimum, and avoided at mealtimes. Exclude alcohol and stop smoking: both compromise the health of the baby and the mother's nutritional status and dramatically increase the risk of miscarriage. If you suffer from allergies (pp. 19–21), avoid known food and chemical allergens as babies can become sensitized while in the womb.

SUPPLEMENTS

Multivitamin and mineral supplement which must contain at least 15 mg zinc, 10 mg vitamin B_6 and 400 mcg folic acid. Take 100 g vitamin C with meals to enhance iron absorption.

For morning sickness, nausea and high blood pressure take extra supplements of vitamin B_6 (30 mg), calcium (500 mg twice daily) and magnesium (250 mg twice daily).

For constipation, haemorrhoids and varicose veins, take extra vitamin C (100 mg) and a bioflavonoid complex (250 mg twice daily) (p. 15).

For postnatal depression, take extra vitamin B-complex, calcium (500 mg twice daily) and magnesium (250 mg twice daily).

HERBAL

Raspberry (p. 43, caution). Drink raspberry leaf tea once daily six weeks prior to delivery to prepare for childbirth.

Fennel. Drink a decoction made from fennel seeds to increase milk flow.

Calendula/Echinacea. Use ointment for sore, chapped nipples and mastitis, or apply a macerated fresh cabbage leaf inside your bra as a poultice.

AROMATHERAPY

Clary sage oil (p. 49, caution). Massage with 5 drops essential oil mixed with 1 tbsp carrier oil once labour has begun – to soothe and ease the pain.

HOMEOPATHY

Arnica. Start taking 30C three times daily two days prior to delivery date. After childbirth take every half hour for the first two hours and then three times daily for two weeks. If you are not breastfeeding, your baby should also receive Arnica to help recover from the shock and trauma of delivery.

BIOCHEMIC TISSUE SALTS

Calc. fluor. four times daily for haemorrhoids and varicose veins

Nat. sulph. four times daily for morning sickness and digestive problems, including dyspepsia

EXERCISE

The mental and physical benefits for both mother and baby of regular aerobic exercise are far-reaching. Physical fitness promotes easier delivery and faster recovery. Walking

TINCTURES

If drinking a herbal tincture add 45 ml (3 tbsp) just-boiled water to the dose and allow to cool before drinking. This ensures that most of the alcohol evaporates.

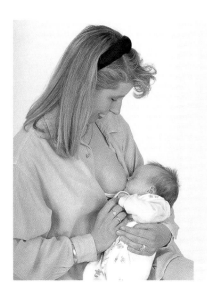

BREAST IS BEST

Breast milk, aside from being a perfect food, is rich in many factors which have profound long-term effects on the development and effectiveness of the child's immune system. The incidence of infections and allergic conditions (such as asthma and eczema) is much reduced in breastfed babies.

and swimming are the best activities. It is also recommended that you attend yoga classes. Practise pelvic floor exercises as often as you can: as hard as you can, squeeze the same muscles which you would use to stop the flow of urine, then relax them. Repeat 20 times. These exercises, done regularly, will help prevent the later development of bladder control problems and uterine prolapse.

ACUPRESSURE

Joining the Valley (LI 4) (p. 73). This point **is not recommended during pregnancy,** but can prove invaluable for labour pain. Apply firm, steady pressure in the direction of the index finger bone for one minute as often as necessary to each hand in turn.

Sea of Energy (CV 6). Stimulate this point (p. 72) three times daily for one minute for several weeks after the birth.

MASSAGE

Regular massage (pp. 74–77) is recommended during pregnancy, after childbirth and for the baby. However, do not massage over any varicose veins.

MIND/BODY

Regular meditation, relaxation activities and positive thinking are recommended as an antidote to the harmful psychological and physical effects of stress (p. 87). Evidence suggests that the unborn baby 'experiences' everything the mother does; whatever relaxes or pleases the mother will do the same for the baby.

CAUTION

♦ It is best to avoid all herbal remedies and essential oils in the first three months of pregnancy, unless professionally advised. Please refer to *Herbal Healing*, pp. 32–45, and *Aromatherapy*, pp. 46–49, for specifics about each herb and essential oil.

♦ Of those herbs recommended throughout this book, the following should be used with caution or avoided during pregnancy: agnus castus, aloe vera, black cohosh, dong quai, feverfew, golden seal, raspberry, sage, and uva ursi. Peppermint may disturb milk flow in nursing mothers.

♦ Clary sage oil (p. 49) is not recommended during pregnancy, but only once labour has begun.

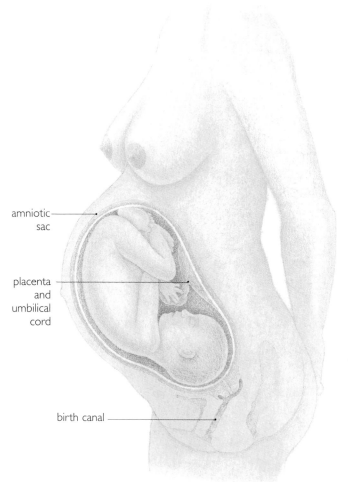

amniotic sac

placenta and umbilical cord

birth canal

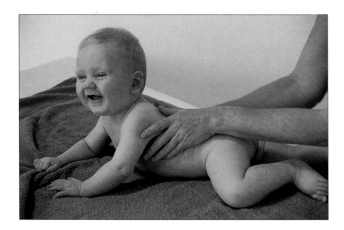

Above: *Touch is crucial to healthy development: babies who are not touched regularly have much higher levels of stress hormones which adversely affect their growth and development.*

Above: *Close to the end of pregnancy, the baby will usually begin to move down into the pelvis in preparation for birth. This is known as lightening or 'engagement'.*

MALE COMPLAINTS

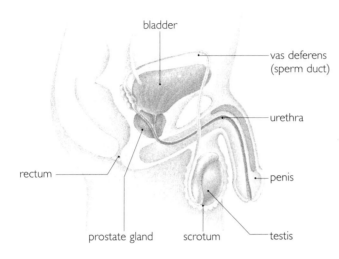

Above: *Male reproductive organs*

PROSTATE PROBLEMS

BENIGN PROSTATIC HYPERTROPHY (BPH) (enlarged prostate gland)

This gland, which surrounds the neck of the bladder, becomes enlarged, causing a progressively worse obstruction of the flow of urine.
SUPPLEMENTS
Zinc 15 mg
Flaxseed 1 tbsp
Phytosterol supplements (p. 14) or
4 tbsp pumpkin seeds daily
HERBAL
Saw palmetto 160 mg standardized extract twice daily

PROSTATITIS (prostate inflammation due to infection)

Chronic prostatitis is difficult to treat, even with antibiotics. The following treatments may help.
SUPPLEMENTS
Multivitamin and minerals
Vitamin C 200 mg twice daily
Zinc 15 mg
HERBAL
Uva ursi (p. 36, caution)
Saw palmetto 160 mg standardized extract twice daily

CHEMICAL DANGERS

Many chemicals used in industry and agriculture contain substances which act as powerful oestrogen mimics and are not easily broken down and excreted. They are associated with the steady decline in male fertility and rise in hormone-dependent cancers such as prostate cancer. Plant phyto-estrogens, widely present in many plant foods, protect the body from the damaging effects of these chemicals.

WARNING

Medical examination is recommended for all problems relating to urination, in order to exclude serious conditions such as cancer of the prostate, sexually transmitted diseases, or kidney disease.

CYSTITIS/URETHRITIS

Infections of the urinary tract are not as common in men as they are in women, as the urethra is much longer in men. Infections are characterized by burning and itching on urination and should be medically investigated.

INFERTILITY

Ten to twenty percent of males reaching maturity in industrialized countries are sub-fertile. Nutritional deficiencies (especially of zinc, selenium, folic acid and vitamin C) and the increasing abundance of chemicals in our environment have been linked to the steady decline in the quantity and quality of human sperm. It is important to give up smoking and caffeine, to reduce alcohol intake and to wear loose underpants and trousers in order to keep the testes cool.
DIET
Eat plenty of fresh fruit, vegetables and pulses, organically grown if possible. Reduce intake of animal fats and processed foods.
SUPPLEMENTS
Multivitamin and mineral supplement
Vitamin C 200 mg twice daily
Vitamin E (p. 26, caution) 400 IU
Zinc 30 mg
Selenium 200 mcg
Flaxseed oil 1 tbsp
Seaweed/algae (p. 25) supplement as directed

CIRCULATORY PROBLEMS

CARDIOVASCULAR DISEASE (CVD)

(This includes diseases of the heart and arteries.) Arteries have the vital function of carrying blood, containing nourishment and oxygen, to tissues throughout the body. The most common cause of death in developed countries is due to a blockage in one of the arteries supplying the heart (a heart attack) or in one supplying the brain (a stroke). The disease begins when LDL cholesterol (p. 15) is deposited inside the arteries. These fatty deposits are oxidized and harden to form plaque, a process called atherosclerosis. As the deposits of plaque grow, the blood flow becomes increasingly restricted and blood clots are more likely to form, leading to a total blockage.

Common symptoms of atherosclerosis include: angina (pain in the chest, throat and left arm after exertion), breathlessness, weakness, dizziness, poor peripheral circulation and reduced mental functioning. However, there are sometimes no warning symptoms, leading to cardiovascular disease being known as 'the silent killer'.

To keep your arteries clear and healthy you have to address and modify the key risk factors: obesity, high

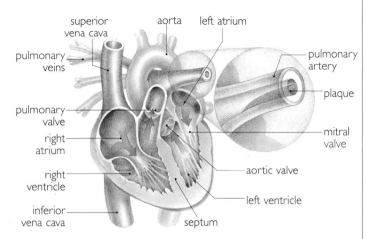

Above: *This cross-section of the heart shows a close-up detail of the build-up of plaque in the pulmonary artery.*

blood pressure, diabetes, high LDL cholesterol levels, high stress levels, lack of exercise, smoking and the contraceptive pill. Smoking increases blood pressure and, like the contraceptive pill, increases the clotting tendency of blood. Suppressed anger and hostility, particularly over long periods of time, appear to increase the risk of developing cardiovascular disease.

DIET

Dietary measures are aimed at reducing high LDL cholesterol levels and high blood pressure and at increasing the protective HDL cholesterol levels. Follow the guidelines for healthy eating (p. 13), paying particular attention to the following points:

- ◆ Reduce salt intake and alcohol consumption and avoid caffeine-containing drinks.
- ◆ Substantially reduce intake of saturated fats, dairy products, meat and poultry.
- ◆ Eat at least six daily servings of fresh fruit and vegetables.
- ◆ Avoid margarine, and use cold-pressed virgin olive oil instead of vegetable oils rich in omega 6 fatty acids, such as safflower, corn and sunflower (these tend to lower both the bad LDL and the beneficial HDL levels).
- ◆ Eat two to three servings a week of fish rich in omega 3 fatty acids.
- ◆ Increase daily intake of foods high in soluble fibre, such as oats, barley and pulses.

OLIVE OIL – A MEDITERRANEAN ELIXIR!

In the average Cretan diet 45% of kilojoules (calories) comes from fat, of which 30% comes from olive oil, yet people from Crete show the lowest incidence of heart disease in Europe! This is because olive oil is high in a monounsaturated fat called oleic acid. This ingredient works selectively to reduce the harmful LDL cholesterol levels and increase the healthy HDL levels.

Other factors in olive oil work to lower blood pressure, thin the blood and reduce the absorption of dietary cholesterol. Olive oil also contains powerful antioxidants.

SUPPLEMENTS
Multivitamin and mineral supplement
Vitamin B complex
Vitamin C 200 mg twice daily
Vitamin E (p. 26, caution) 600 IU
Bioflavonoid complex (p. 15) 250 mg twice daily
Seaweed supplement (p. 25)
Flaxseed oil 1 tbsp and/or fish oil (p. 18, caution) 2 g
HERBAL
Garlic
Hawthorn
Lime blossom
Ginger
Green tea
Gingko
Ginseng (caution, p. 43)
Siberian ginseng
EXERCISE
Regular aerobic exercise (pp. 51–54) modifies many of the key heart disease risk factors by countering the harmful effects of stress and preventing obesity.

RELAXATION
Regular meditation or breathing exercises are recommended to counteract the negative effects of stress.

Left: *Moderate drinking (one to two drinks a day) raises protective HDL cholesterol levels and lowers blood pressure. However, the 'window' of alcohol's benefit is small: if more than this is consumed these beneficial effects are offset by an increase in the risk of death from other causes, particularly cancer. Red wine, rich in bioflavonoids, is the healthiest form of alcohol.*

HEALTHY ARTERIES
Bioflavonoids, particularly the anthocyanidins, proanthocyanidins and catechins, are powerful antioxidants. In combination with vitamins C and E they prevent arterial wall damage and the oxidation of LDL cholesterol which leads to the formation of plaque. They also strengthen and tone blood capillaries. The herbs recommended above are all rich sources of these protective bioflavonoids.

HIGH BLOOD PRESSURE
This often occurs without symptoms and is only discovered during a routine medical checkup. If your blood pressure is between 100/60 and 140/90 it is considered normal. Anything between 140/90 and 160/90 should be addressed by following the advice recommended for cardiovascular disease. Anything over 160/100 requires medical attention.
DIET AND SUPPLEMENTS
Follow the treatment advice for cardiovascular disease and include 500 mg calcium and 500 mg magnesium.

HERBS TO CONTROL BLOOD PRESSURE
Herbal circulation stimulants such as chillis, ginger, cinnamon and hawthorn reduce blood pressure by relaxing and dilating the blood vessels (exercise and relaxation do the same). Stress, caffeine and smoking have the opposite effect – they constrict the blood vessels and force up blood pressure.

Make a cinnamon decoction by bringing 3 cups of water and 30 g (1 oz) dried cinnamon sticks to the boil. Simmer uncovered for 20–30 minutes. Strain, cover and refrigerate. Take one wine-glass dose three times daily between meals for at least four weeks.

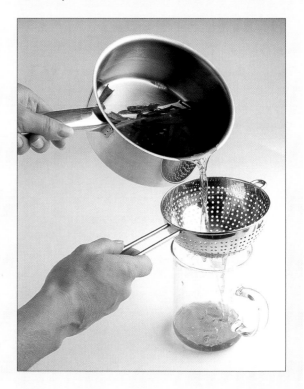

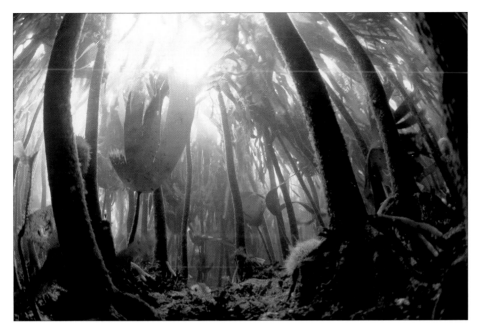

Left: *The Fucus and Laminaria species are the most medicinal seaweeds/algae. Seaweed lowers blood pressure and cholesterol levels, thins the blood and counteracts the harmful effects of high salt consumption. Take these supplements dried, powdered or in tablet form, or use edible seaweeds in cooking.*

VARICOSE VEINS

SUPPLEMENTS
Vitamin C 200 mg twice daily
Bioflavonoid complex (p. 15) 250 mg twice daily
HERBAL
Witch hazel (p. 40, caution). Apply in a cold compress to soothe painful veins.

FLUID RETENTION

Fluid retention is due to an increased volume of fluid within the circulatory system and the leaking of fluid from the blood vessels into surrounding tissues, causing general or localized oedema (swelling). Mild cases are common premenstrually, during pregnancy and after standing or sitting in one position for a long time. If, together with fluid retention, your weight fluctuates substantially, suspect a food allergy (pp. 19–21). Persistent cases must be investigated.

DIET AND SUPPLEMENTS
Follow the advice for cardiovascular disease (pp. 99–100), and ensure that salt and sugar intake is reduced. Eat foods with a natural diuretic action, such as apples, grapes, celery, parsley and asparagus. If necessary, exclude suspected food allergens (pp. 19–21).
HERBAL
Dandelion
Chicory
Gingko

CHILBLAINS

Chilblains, inflamed and swollen patches of skin which burn and itch, are caused by prolonged exposure to cold coupled with poor circulation. Sensitive extremities such as toes, fingers and ears are most at risk and should be well covered in cold weather. Smoking contributes to the problem.

DIET AND SUPPLEMENTS
Follow the advice given for cardiovascular disease (pp. 99–100).
HERBAL
Chilli (p. 39, caution)
Ginger
Cinnamon
Calendula. Apply ointment to affected area twice daily.
AROMATHERAPY
Rosemary oil. Apply a warm compress for 3 minutes, then a cold compress for 1 minute. Alternatively, use cold and warm foot or hand baths. Add 6 drops essential oil to each bath and bathe affected area, alternating as for compresses.

SKIN, HAIR AND NAIL PROBLEMS

SKIN PROBLEMS

PIMPLES/SPOTS

This skin condition affects many people at some stage in their lives. It can have profound psychological and social effects, especially for teenagers.

There are two processes involved – hyperkeratosis and increased sebum (oil) production. In puberty and premenstrually,

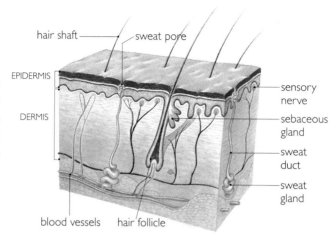

hair shaft — sweat pore

EPIDERMIS

DERMIS

sensory nerve

sebaceous gland

sweat duct

sweat gland

blood vessels   hair follicle

Above: A cross-section of the skin shows unblocked, healthy follicles.

sebaceous production is increased due to an increased production of the adrenal gland hormones (androgen). Sebum is produced in the hair follicles. Cells lining the follicles are continually being shed and replaced. The dead cells mix with the sebum and work their way to the surface where they are washed off. In cases of hyperkeratosis the follicle wall thickens and blocks the movement of the dead cells and sebum to the surface. As more oil is produced, the hair follicle swells, forming a distended pore or blackhead. If it closes over it is known as a whitehead. Certain bacteria will then break down the sebum, resulting in inflammation and the formation of pus – the dreaded full-blown pimple!

Vigorous washing and scrubbing are not recommended – this can increase the production of sebum. Heredity is a strong factor, but the following advice may help. Wash twice a day with a pH-neutral cleanser. Do not use alcohol-based astringents. Light make-up can be used. Do not touch or squeeze the pimples, as this will only spread the infection.

DIET

Diet does not appear to be an important factor. However, many people find their condition worsens after eating sweet and fatty foods, which tend to depress immune function; it thus makes sense to exclude or moderate intake of these. Foods containing iodine (kelp, shellfish, iodized salt, etcetera) may aggravate the condition.

SUPPLEMENTS
Betacarotene 10 mg
Vitamin B complex
Vitamin C 200 mg twice daily
Vitamin E (p. 26, caution) 400 IU
Zinc 15 mg
HERBAL
Garlic
Echinacea
Calendula. Dilute tincture 1:20 with water and apply with cotton wool.
Agnus castus for premenstrual spots
Alpha-hydroxy acid. Apply a 5–12% concentration cream or lotion as directed. Increase concentration gradually if sensitivity is a problem.
AROMATHERAPY
Tea tree or lavender oil. Apply undiluted essential oil to pimple two to three times an hour for acute, painful eruptions, otherwise three times daily.
EXERCISE
Regular aerobic exercise is advised to reduce stress levels, counter any depression about the condition, stimulate immune function and improve skin circulation.

ALLERGIES
A bioflavonoid called quercetin prevents the release of histamine and is useful for treating allergic skin conditions.

ABSCESSES, BOILS AND CARBUNCLES
These are typically caused by a bacterial infection. The first stage is characterized by a painful red swelling, after which pus begins to form. This will usually discharge itself within a few days. Do not squeeze the pus out as this will often spread the infection. (An interconnecting collection of boils is called a carbuncle.)
DIET
Follow the guidelines for healthy eating (p. 13), taking care to include lots of raw vegetables and fruit.

HERBAL
Echinacea
Garlic
Slippery elm. Make a hot paste using slippery elm powder and apply as a poultice. Keep the affected area covered at all times, using chickweed cream or raw honey as a dressing.
HOMEOPATHY
Arsenicum album for hot, burning, painful abscess/boil
Belladonna for abscess/boil which comes up quickly, is very red and painful and throbs violently
Hepar sulph. for recurrent boils
Silica for abscess/boil which is slow to discharge and for those involving a foreign body
Take 30C every 2 hours until it discharges.

ECZEMA/DERMATITIS

Eczema is a type of skin inflammation associated with the formation of red, itchy scales. Sometimes small vesicles form which can burst, causing weeping eczema. The term dermatitis is usually reserved for eczema which has an external cause, such as contact with certain chemicals, perfumes, metals (particularly nickel in metallic watch straps) and plants. Atopic eczema (which affects 3% of all children) is an inherited type which often occurs in conjunction with asthma, hayfever or urticaria. It is due to an immunological defect and the condition has been associated with certain food and environmental allergies (pp. 19–21). If nothing else is available, add ½ cup sodium bicarbonate to bath water for relief.
DIET
The most commonly implicated foods and chemicals are cows' milk, wheat, eggs, fish, sugar and certain food additives. (See pp. 20–21 for advice on exclusion diets.) Exclude fried foods and margarine.
   Fresh green cabbage leaves (liquidized or pounded) applied to the affected areas and covered with a bandage may bring dramatic relief.
SUPPLEMENTS
Multivitamin and mineral supplement
Vitamin C 200 mg twice daily
Quercetin 400 mg twice daily between meals
Zinc 15 mg
Flaxseed oil 1 tbsp

SKIN INFLAMMATION

Blend three fresh, washed cabbage leaves, rich in quercetin, with 50 ml distilled witch hazel and apply twice daily to all inflammatory skin conditions.

Borage oil (p. 17) 500 mg twice daily
Phytosterol supplement (p. 14)
HERBAL
Echinacea
Stinging nettle
Echinacea or rooibos. Take internally and apply to affected areas.
Calendula, chickweed or aloe vera.
Apply ointment or extract to affected areas regularly.
AROMATHERAPY
Lavender or chamomile oil. Use in a cold compress.

WARTS AND VERUCCAS (viral)
HERBAL/AROMATHERAPY
Garlic oil or tea tree oil. Apply fresh garlic juice or tea tree oil to affected area and cover with an airtight plaster/dressing. Repeat twice daily.

FUNGAL INFECTIONS

All moist areas of the body are susceptible to fungal infections. The tinea fungus is responsible for ringworm, athlete's foot, Dhobie's itch (in the groin) and some finger and toenail infections. Others are due to Candida albicans.
DIET
To ensure a permanent cure for all persistent fungal infections, follow the guidelines for healthy eating (p. 13). Exclude refined foods, sugar and alcohol.
SUPPLEMENTS
Multivitamin and mineral supplement
Vitamin B complex
Zinc 15 mg
Vitamin C 200 mg twice daily
HERBAL
Calendula. Apply ointment twice daily.
Garlic. Apply freshly squeezed juice twice daily.
AROMATHERAPY
Tea tree oil. Apply 5 drops essential oil mixed with 1 tbsp carrier oil twice daily.

GENERAL ADVICE FOR HAIR, NAIL AND SKINCARE

All skin problems will benefit from following the guidelines for healthy eating (p. 13), taking a multivitamin and mineral supplement, extra vitamin C (200 mg twice daily), zinc (15 mg) and a bioflavonoid complex (250 mg twice daily), and adding 1 tbsp of flaxseed oil to the diet daily. Brewer's yeast (10–15 tablets daily) is an excellent natural vitamin B complex supplement for all skin, hair and nail conditions, but is not recommended for people with a yeast allergy or chronic candidiasis. It is also beneficial to take regular exercise.

Dandruff

Most cases of dandruff are due to a fungal infection. Fresh lemon juice or cider vinegar (diluted with water in a 1:20 ratio) rubbed into the scalp 30 minutes prior to washing can be very effective, especially if the scalp is itchy. Follow the general advice above (see box).

AROMATHERAPY

Rosemary oil. Massage 10 drops essential oil mixed with 2 tbsp carrier oil into scalp and leave for 2 hours before washing. Add 5 drops rosemary oil to the final rinsing water.

HERPES INFECTIONS
Herpes simplex (cold sores and genital herpes)

This virus often produces no symptoms on first infection. However, it stays dormant in the nerve fibres, sporadically erupting when resistance is low due to nutrient deficiency, disease or stress. Type 1 Herpes simplex virus (HSV) is the most common kind and produces cold sores around the mouth and nose. Type 2 HSV causes painful blisters on the genital organs. Both types can be transmitted during the active phase of the virus by close contact such as kissing or sexual intercourse.

DIET

Follow the guidelines for healthy eating (p. 13). During the active phase avoid peanuts, seeds, chocolate and cereals, as these are rich in arginine, an amino acid which favours the growth of the herpes simplex virus.

SUPPLEMENTS

Vitamin B complex

Vitamin C 200 mg three times daily

Zinc 15 mg (Also apply zinc salve directly to affected area.)

L-lysine (amino acid supplement) 500–1 000 mg daily on an empty stomach

HERBAL

St John's wort (p. 40, caution), echinacea or garlic. Apply directly to affected area.

AROMATHERAPY

Tea tree oil. Apply 5 drops essential oil mixed with 1 tbsp carrier oil every 2 hours as soon as the infection begins to develop.

HOMEOPATHY

Nat. mur.

Take 30C every 2 hours until relief is obtained.

RELAXATION

Stress is known to be a strong contributory factor in the development of herpes. Adopt a regular programme of relaxation (pp. 83–84) and aerobic exercise (pp. 50–53).

Herpes zoster (shingles)

This condition is caused by a reactivated chickenpox virus and is characterized by a painful blistered rash which typically develops on one side of the chest or back. If it occurs on the forehead, medical help should be sought immediately as this may lead to eye damage. Pain can be experienced for many months or even years after the rash has cleared. Stress is a strong precipitating factor and should be addressed.

SUPPLEMENTS

Vitamin E (p. 26, caution) 400 IU

Zinc 15 mg

HERBAL

St John's wort (p. 40, caution). Take internally. In addition apply diluted tincture in a cold compress.

Chilli (p. 39, caution). Apply capsaicin cream to affected area.

AROMATHERAPY

Tea tree oil. Apply in a cold compress to affected area.

HOMEOPATHY

Rhus tox.

Hypericum

Take 30C every few hours while symptoms are intense.

PSORIASIS

Psoriasis is characterized by patches of rapidly dividing skin cells which do not form a proper outer layer and result in well-defined red plaques covered in silvery scales. Salt baths (1 kg [2¼ lb] salt in warm bath water) and careful exposure to sunlight will help clear the condition. Stress may precipitate an attack.

DIET

Reduce intake of animal fats and increase that of fresh vegetables, fruit, brown rice and fish rich in omega 3 fatty acids. Eliminate alcohol and margarine as they interfere with essential fatty acid metabolism. Oatmeal or cooked porridge poultices and preparations containing vitamin D_3 have an anti-inflammatory effect.

SUPPLEMENTS

Multivitamin and mineral supplement

Vitamin E (p. 26, caution) 400 IU

Zinc 15 mg

Flaxseed oil 1 tbsp or fish oil (p. 18, caution) 2 g

Phytosterol supplement (p. 14)

HERBAL

Golden seal (p. 40, caution)

Echinacea

AROMATHERAPY

Lavender, sandalwood (if the affected area is very dry) or German chamomile oil. Massage 10 drops essential oil mixed with 2 tbsp carrier oil into affected areas (or add to bath water).

HOMEOPATHY

Arsenicum album for dry, rough, scaly skin which is worse with cold and better with heat.

Graphites for dry, cracking skin with sticky, honey-like discharge

Petroleum for dry, cracked, itchy skin with thin, watery discharges

Sulphur for red, intensely itchy and burning skin where symptoms are worse with heat and after washing

Take in the 6C potency three times daily for 4 weeks.

SCAR TISSUE/KELOID GROWTH

SUPPLEMENTS

Vitamin C 200 mg three times daily

Vitamin E (p. 26, caution) 600 IU

Zinc 15 mg

HERBAL

Witch hazel (p. 40, caution). Apply distilled witch hazel to wounds to prevent scarring.

HOMEOPATHY

Graphites for keloid growth

Take 6C potency three times daily for 4 weeks.

MASSAGE

Regular massage with a lubricant containing vitamin E is one of the best ways of healing scar tissue.

DRY SKIN

Follow the general advice for hair, nail and skincare (p. 104). Add 1 cup cider vinegar to bath water to relieve dryness, and use cocoa butter as an excellent skin emollient.

AROMATHERAPY

Sandalwood oil. Add 6 drops essential oil to bath water, or massage with 10 drops essential oil mixed with 2 tbsp avocado oil/olive oil.

GREASY SKIN

(See advice for pimples/spots on p. 102.) Apply tomato pulp or fresh lemon juice to oily areas for 15 minutes and wash off, then apply a lotion made with 2 tbsp distilled witch hazel (p. 40, caution) mixed with 10 drops lavender oil.

AGE SPOTS

These are believed to result, in part, from free radical damage to the skin. Follow the general skincare advice (p. 104). Lemon juice, buttermilk, sour milk or natural live yoghurt are all gentle bleaches: apply at least twice daily. Alpha-hydroxy acid preparations (in a 10–15% concentration) can also be used.

ALPHA-HYDROXY ACIDS

Alpha-hydroxy acids, a class of acids found in many everyday foods such as fruit and cultured milk products, stimulate cell renewal, moisturize dry skin, improve skin elasticity and tone, reduce the appearance of fine lines, lighten pigmentation and reduce the hyperkeratosis of follicles responsible for spots and pimples. Improvements are seen within six weeks, and alpha-hydroxy preparations should be used indefinitely for maximum benefits.

SOLAR KERATOSIS

These pre-cancerous lesions are characterized by rough, scaly inflamed patches which never seem to heal. Follow the general advice for hair, nail and skincare (p. 104).

HERBAL

Green tea. Drink infusion; apply preparations containing an extract of green tea to affected areas.

URTICARIA/NETTLE RASH

This very itchy and patchy rash is usually caused by an allergic reaction to something in the environment or something eaten. It can also occur after exercise or intense emotion.

GENERAL

Follow recommendations for eczema (p. 103).

HOMEOPATHY

Aconite if brought on by intense emotion

Urtica urens if intensely itchy and burning

Rhus tox. if accompanied by extreme restlessness

Take 30C of chosen remedy every 30 minutes until relief is obtained.

HAIR PROBLEMS

Hair problems may be due to nutritional deficiencies, hormonal imbalances, hereditary factors, stress, harsh treatments involving heat and chemicals and various drugs. Follow the general advice for hair, nail and skincare (p. 104).

AROMATHERAPY

Rosemary oil. Add 3–4 drops essential oil to final rinsing water if you have dark hair.

Chamomile oil. Add 3–4 drops essential oil to final rinsing water if you have fair hair.

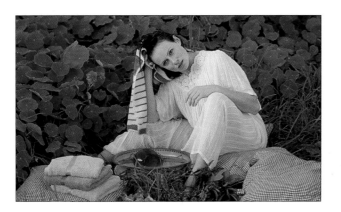

HAIR LOSS

Sudden hair loss may be the result of stress and shock and should be treated appropriately. Mixtures which are applied topically and contain biotin and niacin (vitamin B_3) or herbal mixtures containing Jaborandi may reduce hair loss. Follow the general advice for hair, nail and skincare (see p. 104).

HERBAL

Dong quai (p. 36, caution), black cohosh (p. 39, caution), agnus castus (p. 44, caution), Sage (p. 43, caution) if hair loss is associated with recent pregnancy or menopause

DRY HAIR

Massage 2 tbsp warmed olive oil into the scalp and hair and cover with a hot, wet towel for 20 minutes (reheat the towel as soon as it cools). Shampoo as usual.

GREASY HAIR

After washing hair, rinse with the juice of one lemon and warm water, or add ½ cup cider vinegar to final rinsing water.

NAIL PROBLEMS

Many nail problems are due to skin diseases such as eczema and psoriasis or fungal or bacterial infections. These should be treated appropriately. Prolonged immersion in water may lead to brittle and split nails. Nail quality is affected by various nutrient deficiencies, especially of iron, zinc, calcium and fatty acids. Iron deficiency leads to a thinning of the nail. The shape of the nail may also change from a normal downward curve to become flat or even upturned (spoon shaped). White spots on the nails are often a sign of zinc deficiency. Brittle, ridged nails may be a sign of calcium deficiency. Follow the general advice for hair, nail and skincare (see p. 104).

SUPPLEMENTS (EXTRA)

Betacarotene 10 mg

Calcium 250 mg twice daily

Borage oil (p. 17, caution) 500 mg twice daily

Left: *Rosemary is the best known herb for creating beautiful hair. Add 4 drops essential oil to rinsing water to stimulate circulation and improve hair growth, lustre and scalp condition.*

EAR, NOSE AND THROAT PROBLEMS

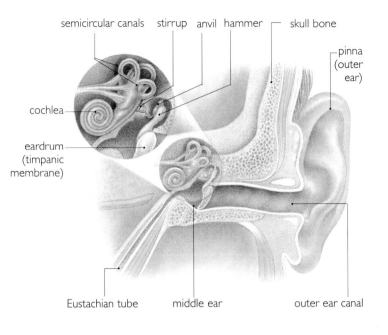

semicircular canals   stirrup   anvil hammer   skull bone

pinna (outer ear)

cochlea

eardrum (timpanic membrane)

Eustachian tube   middle ear   outer ear canal

Above: *A cross-section of the ear showing the outer ear, the middle ear and the remarkable inner ear structures.*

EAR PROBLEMS

DEAFNESS

Temporary deafness may be due to a build-up of wax in the outer ear, a foreign object in the ear (especially in a child), a chronic ear infection or a cold. Wax or foreign objects should be cleared by a trained practitioner. Never poke about in the ear. Treatments for deafness due to an ear infection or a cold can be found under the appropriate sections. Hearing may also be impaired by poor nutrition and the ageing process.

DIET
Follow the guidelines for healthy eating (p. 13).
SUPPLEMENTS
Multivitamin and mineral supplement
Vitamin C 200 mg twice daily
Vitamin E (p. 26, caution) 600 IU
Bioflavonoid complex (p. 15) 250 mg twice daily
HERBAL
Ginkgo

TINNITUS

This distressing condition is common in older people and is characterized by incessant noise (buzzing, ringing, hissing or whistling) in the ears. Follow the advice given for deafness (see below left).

EARACHE

This may be caused by an outer or a middle ear infection. (It also may be associated with sinusitis, toothache, catarrh and mumps.)
HERBAL
St John's wort or garlic oil. For outer ear infection put 3 drops oil in ear and cover with plug of cotton wool. Hold a hot water bottle against painful ear.

NOSE AND THROAT PROBLEMS

CATARRH

Catarrh, as a general term, describes the discharge from inflamed mucous membranes, particularly those lining the nose and sinuses. See sinusitis (pp. 108–109) and hayfever/chronic allergic rhinitis (p. 119).

GINGIVITIS

This is a bacterial infection of the gums often caused by a build-up of plaque. Teeth should be brushed and flossed regularly. Sprinkle salt on a toothbrush and use instead of toothpaste.
HERBAL
Green/black tea. Gargle with the infusion and then swallow.
Sage. Gargle three times daily with infusion or 3 drops sage oil in ¼ cup water. Do not swallow.

TEA
Tea, especially green tea, is the perfect herb for dental health. It is active against the bacteria that cause plaque and abscesses and is a rich source of fluoride. Halitosis, often caused by dental disease, can be effectively treated with tea.

MOUTH ULCERS

These painful raw spots may be due to injury or spicy, acidic or sweet foods. They are sometimes caused by substances in toothpaste. Try to identify and avoid offending foods. Sprinkle salt on a toothbrush and use instead of toothpaste.

HERBAL

Sage. Gargle three times daily with infusion or 3 drops sage oil in ¼ cup water. Do not swallow.

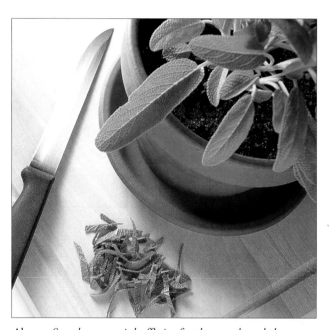

Above: *Sage has a special affinity for the mouth and throat.*

ORAL THRUSH

This is caused by the Candida albicans yeast and results in painful white patches in the mouth. It often develops after antibiotic treatment and is associated with a weakened immune system. See candidiasis (p. 130).

HERBAL

Calendula. Gargle with an infusion or diluted tincture (1 tsp to ¼ cup water) three times daily and swallow.

AROMATHERAPY

Tea tree oil. Gargle with 2 drops essential oil in ¼ cup water, or dab essential oil on affected areas. Do not swallow.

SINUSITIS

The sinuses are small cavities in the skull bones around the eyes and above the nose. The membranes lining these cavities can become inflamed and full of mucus owing to infection or irritation (from house dust, tobacco smoke and so on). Chronic sinusitis may be related to a food allergy, particularly to dairy products. Emotional stress may exacerbate the condition and should be treated with Bach flower remedies (pp. 64–67) and a relaxation programme (pp. 83–84).

DIET AND SUPPLEMENTS

Follow the advice given for sore throats (opposite).

HERBAL

Garlic

Chilli (p. 39, caution)

Echinacea

Golden seal (p. 40, caution)

AROMATHERAPY

Eucalyptus oil. Use 2 drops essential oil in a bowl of boiling water as a steam inhalation. Gently massage painful areas with small circular movements as you breathe the vapour.

Below: *A warm to hot compress placed across the sinuses can be a very effective way to relieve blocked, painful sinuses.*

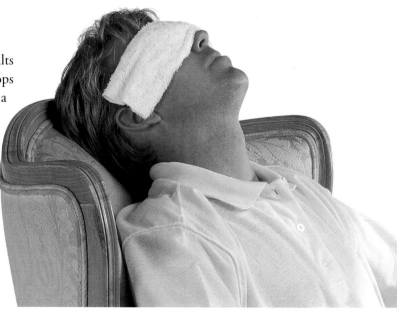

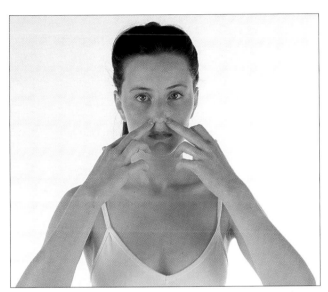

Above: *The Welcoming Perfume (LI 20) points are located just to the side of each nostril.*

ACUPRESSURE

Welcoming Perfume (LI 20). Stimulate both points for several minutes every half hour to relieve sinus pain.

SNORING

Obesity, alcohol and smoking all worsen this condition, which is more prevalent in men (who tend to carry excess weight around their necks). Adequate weight loss is the most effective cure.

RELAXATION

Practise the breathing exercises suggested on p. 84 before you go to sleep, and try not to sleep on your back.

SORE THROATS (including those due to laryngitis, pharyngitis and tonsillitis)

It is essential for adults who suffer recurrent bouts of laryngitis to stop smoking and reduce alcohol consumption.

Recurrent tonsillitis in a child may indicate the presence of a food allergy (pp. 19–21) or stress. Bach flower remedies (pp. 64–67) should be given if stress is an underlying problem, especially for children.

DIET

If the sore throat is accompanied by a fever, fast for 24 hours and drink plenty of filtered or mineral water.

Break the fast with lightly steamed vegetables, salad and brown rice. If there is no fever, follow the guidelines for healthy eating (p. 13), taking care to exclude refined carbohydrates (especially sugar) and dairy products and to reduce intake of animal fats. Eat fresh pineapple, which has an anti-inflammatory effect.

SUPPLEMENTS

Multivitamin and mineral supplement

Vitamin C 200 mg three times daily

Zinc gluconate lozenges to be sucked twice daily, or take zinc tablets (15 mg)

Flaxseed oil 1 tbsp

HERBAL

Ginger

Garlic

Echinacea

Astragalus if you suffer from repeated infections

AROMATHERAPY

Eucalyptus oil (p. 49, caution). Apply in a cold compress to the throat.

HOMEOPATHY

Aconite for hot, dry sore throat which comes on suddenly, often at night

Belladonna for painful, throbbing throat accompanied by a flushed face and fever

Hepar sulph. for painful throat which feels as if something is stuck inside

Mercurius for painful, raw throat and unpleasant breath

Take 30C of chosen remedy every 30 minutes until relief is obtained.

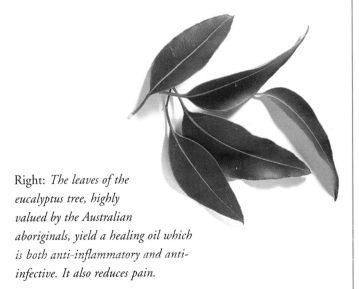

Right: *The leaves of the eucalyptus tree, highly valued by the Australian aboriginals, yield a healing oil which is both anti-inflammatory and anti-infective. It also reduces pain.*

EYE PROBLEMS

CONJUNCTIVITIS AND STYES

The conjunctiva, a delicate membrane covering the whites of the eyes and the inside of the lids, may become inflamed due to an infection, an allergic reaction (see hayfever) or from various irritants such as tobacco smoke and ultraviolet light (arc eye). The affected eyes should not be touched or rubbed and, in the case of infection, strict hygiene must be observed. A stye is an infection of a sebaceous gland at the root of an eyelash.

HERBAL
Calendula. Bathe eyes with an infusion.
Alternatively, place used, warm, ordinary tea bags firmly on closed eyes and leave for 10 minutes.

CATARACTS, BLURRED VISION, EYE STRAIN, TIRED EYES, NEAR-SIGHTEDNESS AND CHRONIC CONJUNCTIVITIS

DIET
Eat plenty of fresh fruit and vegetables in order to supply adequate quantities of the antioxidant carotenoids lutein and zeanxanthin, which specifically target and protect the eyes.

SUPPLEMENTS
Multivitamin and mineral supplement
Vitamin C 200 mg twice daily
Vitamin E (p. 26, caution) 600 IU

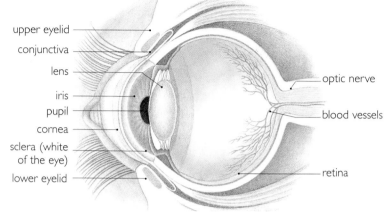

Above: *A cross-section of the eye.*

HERBAL
Bilberry/blueberry

ACUPRESSURE
Third Eye (GV 24.5). Close your eyes and gently apply pressure to this point for one minute several times a day.

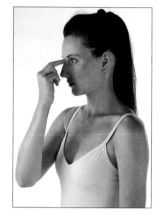

EXERCISE
The Bates Method is a set of exercises designed by New York eye specialist William Bates to naturally strengthen the muscles that control each eye. Practised regularly, they can help anyone with eye strain, tired eyes, a mild squint, astigmatism and near- and long-sightedness, even allowing many people to give up wearing glasses. The exercises should be done in a relaxed way without staring and without optical aids.

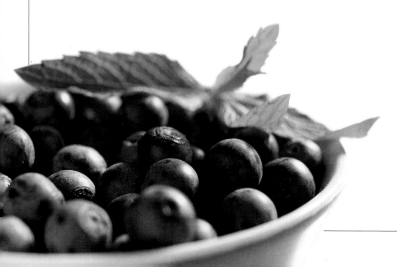

Left: *Bilberries (blueberries) are high in anthocyanidins. These antioxidant flavonoid compounds protect the eye from the damaging effects of free radicals which contribute to cataract formation and deteriorating vision. Bilberry extract improves blood flow to the eyes. It increases the range of vision and enhances the eye's ability to focus, thereby improving image definition. Blurred vision, eye strain and near-sightedness are also helped.*

BATES METHOD

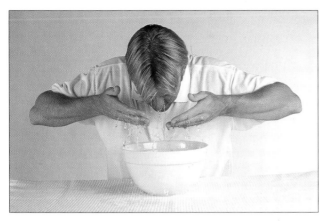

Above: *First thing in the morning, splash closed eyes several times with warm water then several times with cold. Last thing at night do the same in the reverse order. This stimulates blood circulation to the eyes.*

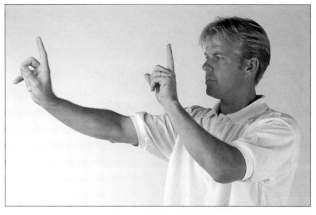

Above: *Practise focusing near and far. Hold one index finger about 10 cm (4 in) from your face and the other finger directly behind it but at arm's length. Focus with both eyes first on one finger and then on the other. Blink between each different focus. Repeat several times. Practise whenever you have a spare moment.*

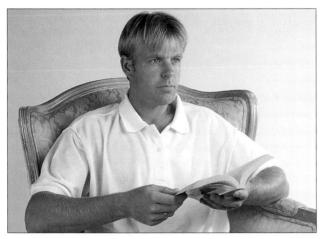

Above: *Avoid staring fixedly at one object for any length of time. When reading, look up and briefly focus elsewhere between pages.*

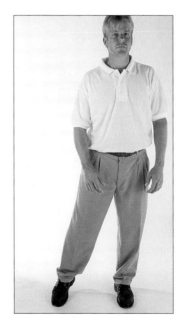

Left: *Stand with your feet apart and gently swing your body from side to side. Let your eyes relax and move with your body. Blink regularly (at least every 10 seconds) to clean and lubricate the eyes.*

NOTE
Always read and watch television in good light.

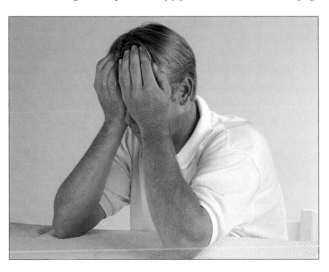

Left: *With your elbows resting on a table or desk, cup your hands and place them over your eyes (without touching them). Relax totally for 10 minutes. This is called palming and should be done twice a day. When using a computer it is recommended that you 'palm' for one minute out of every twelve. Use this quiet period to visualize objects or details such as colours and textures. (Bates believed it was important to practise visualization techniques.)*

PSYCHOLOGICAL AND NEUROLOGICAL PROBLEMS

MENTAL HEALTH REGIME

This regime is indicated for addiction, eating disorders, anxiety syndromes, depression, fatigue, insomnia and dementia. If no improvement is experienced within ten days, suspect a food allergy (pp. 19–21) or chronic candidiasis (p. 130).

DIET

Follow the basic guidelines for healthy eating (p. 13), taking particular care to eat regular meals and to exclude all caffeine and alcohol.

SUPPLEMENTS

Multivitamin and mineral supplement

Vitamin B complex

Vitamin C 200 mg twice daily

Zinc 15 mg

Flaxseed oil 1 tbsp

HERBAL

Ginseng (p. 43, caution)/Siberian ginseng

EXERCISE AND RELAXATION

Stress is a contributory factor to many psychological symptoms and must be addressed. Exercise (pp. 50–55) and meditation (pp. 80–82) are two of the most effective ways of counteracting its damaging effects.

BACH

Choose the appropriate flower remedy to suit your personality and emotional state.

Below: Flower remedies can be used to treat mental problems successfully.

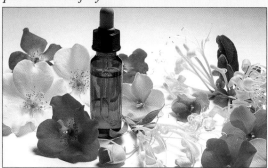

TOBACCO ADDICTION

Most smokers want to stop, but of the more than 30% that try each year less than 3% succeed. Withdrawal symptoms, which include anxiety, irritability, lack of concentration, disturbed sleep and constant cravings, thwart many triers. The use of nicotine patches or gum appears to double the chance of success. Hypnosis and acupuncture help with willpower problems and withdrawal symptoms respectively. The vitamin C supplements recommended in the mental health regime (see left) are critical, as most smokers are deficient in this vitamin; deficiency symptoms include apathy and depression, making it that much harder to give up smoking. Correcting this is the first step in curing this addiction.

GENERAL

Follow the mental health regime (left).

HERBAL

St John's wort (p. 40, caution) to help control withdrawal symptoms

SMOKING

Nicotine is a stimulating drug that provides a temporary lift, but the health price paid by the smoker and those surrounding him or her far exceeds the psychological benefits. The worst effects of smoking are due not to nicotine, however, but to the thousands of harmful substances found in smoke, ranging from tar to cadmium and carbon monoxide. Inhaling cigarette smoke, both actively and passively, is associated with an increased incidence of chronic bronchitis, emphysema, heart disease, high blood pressure and cancer of the lungs, mouth, throat, larynx, pancreas, bladder and cervix. As well as reducing the quality of life of both the smoker and those around who are forced to breathe 'secondary' smoke, smoking reduces the smoker's life by an average of 12 years.

ANOREXIA AND BULIMIA

All eating disorders can be serious and should be handled professionally. Zinc deficiency has been implicated in the development of these disorders.
GENERAL
Follow the mental health regime (p. 112).

ANXIETY AND PANIC ATTACKS

These are often associated with depression, fatigue and insomnia as part of a 'stress' syndrome. Nutritional deficiencies are commonly responsible and correcting these should be the first line of treatment. Caffeine can cause or aggravate these conditions, so exclude all sources.
GENERAL
Follow the mental health regime (p. 112).
HERBAL
St John's wort (p. 40, caution)
ACUPRESSURE
Sea of Tranquility (CV 17). Stimulate several times a day to help relieve anxiety, fear and depression.

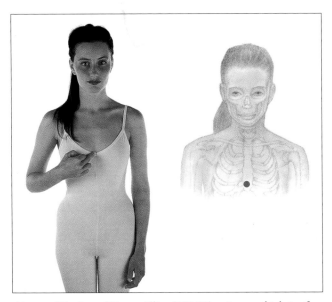

Above: *The Sea of Tranquillity (CV 17) point – which is often tender – is located in the middle of the breastbone, about three fingerwidths up from the bottom of the bone.*

BACH
Rescue Remedy
RELAXATION
Practise the breathing relaxation technique (p. 84) as soon as you start to feel anxious.

DEPRESSION

GENERAL
Follow the mental health regime (p. 112), making sure to include regular exercise, which is particularly effective in improving most cases of mild to moderate depression.
HERBAL
St John's Wort (p. 40, caution)
Lemon balm
Vervain (p. 44, caution)

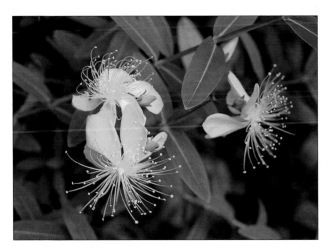

Above: *St John's wort is very effective in managing mild to moderate depression, anxiety and insomnia. This herb compares favourably with many antidepressant drugs and has the added advantage of being without serious side-effects. It works by keeping serotonin (a neurotransmitter known as the 'calming chemical') circulating in the brain. St John's wort may take 6–8 weeks to have an effect.*

AGORAPHOBIA

Agoraphobia is a condition in which sufferers fear leaving a place of safety. When they have to go out they may experience inexplicable panic attacks with palpitations, breathing difficulties, dizziness and increased sweating. One study of sufferers found that all were deficient in one or more of the B vitamins. Over 80% improved dramatically after taking appropriate supplements.

INSOMNIA

DIET
Follow the mental health regime (p. 112), taking care to exclude all caffeine-containing drinks, foods and medications. Milky drinks (especially those made from low fat milk) do not encourage sleep, so avoid them close to bedtime. Honey (p. 90, caution) (1–2 tsp) or sugar added to a sedating herbal tea will encourage sleep by stimulating the production of serotonin.

SUPPLEMENTS
Calcium 1 000 mg
Magnesium 1 000 mg before bedtime

HERBAL
St John's wort (p. 40, caution)
Californian poppy

AROMATHERAPY
Lavender oil. Add 5–10 drops essential oil to bath water or sprinkle on a handkerchief and place on your pillow. Alternatively, massage back with 10 drops mixed with 2 tbsp carrier oil.

HOMEOPATHY
Coffea if you are wide awake with an active mind
Arnica if you are physically and mentally overtired and restless, and the bed feels too hard
Take 30C an hour before and upon going to bed.

EXERCISE
Regular aerobic exercise will help relieve insomnia.

HERBS TO CALM AND SOOTHE
Take the following as regular infusions or in other forms as directed.
- St John's wort for depression, anxiety and insomnia
  - Lime blossom (linden) for anxiety
  - Californian poppy for insomnia
  - Chamomile for insomnia
  - Lemon balm for depression
  - Vervain for depression
  - Wood betony for tension
  - Lavender for tension
  - Redbush for tension

GRIEF

Grief is a natural process to deal with the loss of loved ones. It can be helped by the following gentle remedies.

BACH
Rescue Remedy four times a day for the first few days

HOMEOPATHY
Ignatia for the first stages if you feel weepy and very emotional
Nat. mur. if you prefer to be alone and do not want to be consoled
Staphysagria if you feel angry at what has happened and emotionally on edge
Take 30C three times a day for as long as necessary.

ALZHEIMER'S DISEASE/DEMENTIA

Aluminium status must be assessed because of the neurotoxic nature of this metal (p. 25). Avoid aluminium cookware and any deodorants and antacids which contain aluminium. Vitamin C, calcium and magnesium inhibit aluminium absorption from food and can help reduce body levels of aluminium.

GENERAL
Follow the mental health regime (p. 112).

SUPPLEMENTS (EXTRA)
Vitamin E (p. 26, caution) 600 IU
Calcium 500 mg three times daily
Magnesium 250 mg three times daily
Bioflavonoid complex (p. 15) 250 mg twice daily

HERBAL
Ginkgo

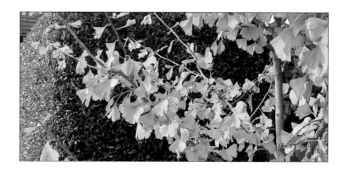

Above: *Gingko biloba, a remedy used for the treatment of age-related diseases, contains a group of highly active flavonoids which are powerful antioxidants capable of protecting against and reversing free radical damage in the brain and throughout the body.*

DYSLEXIA

Many sufferers have been found to have a zinc deficiency and defective essential fatty acid metabolism. If a child also has several of the symptoms listed under hyperactivity (p. 92) then a food allergy should be suspected. Specialized tuition, especially if started early, can dramatically help sufferers.

GENERAL
Follow the mental health regime (p. 112).

DIET
Exclude food allergy as a cause (pp. 19–21).

SUPPLEMENTS (EXTRA)
Fish oil (p. 18, caution) 2 g. If no improvement is experienced after 4 weeks, try borage oil (p. 17, caution) 1 000 mg.

HEADACHES

Most headaches are caused by tension in the scalp, jaw, neck and shoulder muscles as a result of stress coupled with bad posture. Persistent headaches must be medically investigated.

DIET
Exclude caffeine, which can increase muscle tension and anxiety.

SUPPLEMENTS
Flaxseed oil 1 tbsp daily

HERBAL
Wood betony (caution, p. 43) or lavender
Chilli (caution, p. 39) for cluster headaches

ACUPRESSURE
Gates of Consciousness (GB 20). Stimulate both points for two minutes several times an hour until relief is obtained.

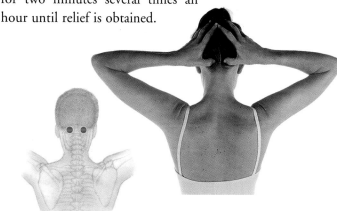

Above: *The Gates of Consciousness (GB 20) points are located in the hollows just below the base of the skull, on either side of the main neck muscles.*

MASSAGE
Use the head and shoulder massage techniques (p. 77) to relieve tension. Massage temples with undiluted lavender or rosemary oil.

PERFECTING YOUR POSTURE

Hold your head up high with neck straight, chin parallel to the ground and shoulders relaxed (below left), instead of carrying your head too far forward from your spine (below centre). The latter position puts extra strain on the neck and shoulder muscles.

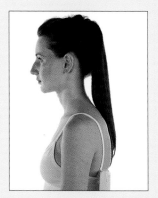

Correct posture

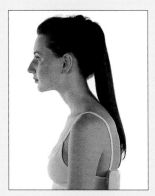

Incorrect posture

When sitting for long periods, exercise your neck several times a day by pulling your chin in as close as you can towards your neck without bending your head or hunching your shoulders. Keep your eyes looking straight ahead. Hold for a minute, relax and repeat 10 times.

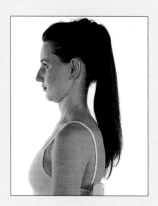

Neck exercise

MIGRAINES

These are severe, often one-sided headaches which are usually accompanied by one or more of the following symptoms: visual disturbances, numbness, tingling and nausea. Food allergy (pp. 19–21) is a significant cause of frequent childhood migraines (over 90% of child migraine sufferers recovered on restricted diets).

DIET

Exclude the following precipitating factors: smoking, the contraceptive pill, caffeine (also present in cola drinks and chocolate), alcohol (especially red wine) and sugar. If this does not help, try to exclude the following items as well: dairy products (especially cheese), wheat, yeast-containing products, chocolate, liver, sausages, broad beans, pickled herrings, oranges, bananas and food additives (especially tartrazine and MSG).

SUPPLEMENTS

Multivitamin and mineral supplement
Vitamin B_6 50 mg
Vitamin C 200 mg twice daily
Vitamin E (p. 26, caution) 400 IU
Magnesium 200 mg
Flaxseed oil 1 tbsp or fish oil (p. 18, caution) 2 g

HERBAL

Feverfew (p. 44, caution), taken regularly, may reduce the frequency and severity of attacks.
Ginger

ACUPRESSURE AND MASSAGE

As for headaches (p. 115)

MIGRAINES EXPLAINED

It has been discovered that blood platelets in migraine sufferers spontaneously 'clump' or stick together preceding an attack. A range of foods and additives (especially milk and tartrazine in children) seem to trigger this reaction, which is, in turn, linked to the release of certain chemicals implicated in the development of a migraine. Nutritional supplements and herbs which have a powerful anticoagulant effect, such as vitamins B_6, C and E, omega 3 fatty acids, feverfew and ginger, help by preventing the platelets from sticking together.

NOTE: If your diet has been totally free of caffeine, a strong cup of coffee can be very effective, in certain cases, in aborting a migraine attack.

NEURALGIA

This condition describes any paroxysmal pain originating in a nerve. Trigeminal neuralgia is confined to the sensory nerve of the face. It is an age-related problem characterized by an increasing frequency of agonizing attacks. Cold draughts, touch or water on the affected area, which is usually very sensitive, can precipitate an attack.

HERBAL

St John's wort (p. 40, caution). Take internally and apply cream or oil to affected area.
Chilli (p. 39, caution). Apply capsaicin cream up to six times a day until pain is relieved.

HOMEOPATHY

Mag. phos. ´ for severe neuralgic pain brought on by cold water, draughts or touch
Take 30C every 10 minutes until relief is obtained.

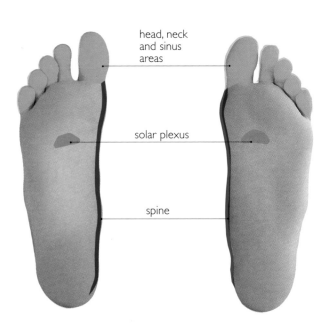

head, neck and sinus areas

solar plexus

spine

Left: For the relief of migraines and headaches, use your thumb tips to apply brief but firm pressure to all the shaded areas in the manner described on p. 73.

RESPIRATORY PROBLEMS

ASTHMA

Asthma is an inflammatory disease of the airways which has a strong allergic basis. Asthma attacks can be triggered by one or more of the following: environmental allergens (such as house dust or airborne pollutants), ingested allergens (such as foods, food additives or drugs), emotional stress, infection, physical activity and sudden temperature changes. It is essential to try to discover the main precipitating factors so that you can modify your environment and lifestyle accordingly.

If the asthma is associated with eczema, urticaria, hayfever and behavioural problems, suspect a food or chemical allergy. Commonly implicated substances are dairy products, eggs, wheat, sugar, yeast, fish (especially shellfish) and various chemical additives (tartrazine [E102], benzoates [E210–219] and sulphites [E220–227]). It is more common to have multiple rather than single food allergies (pp. 19–21).

> **CAUTION** Self-treatment of asthma should be used only in mild, stabilized conditions. Medication must never be stopped suddenly, but phased out gradually with professional guidance and assistance.

DIET
Follow the guidelines for healthy eating (p. 13), taking care to reduce intake of sugar and dairy products and increase intake of fruit and vegetables. If allergy is suspected, exclude suspected allergens (pp. 19–21)

SUPPLEMENTS
Multivitamin and mineral supplement
Vitamin B_6 50 mg
Vitamin C 200 mg twice daily
Quercetin 400 mg twice daily between meals
Flaxseed oil 1 tbsp and/or
fish oil (p. 18, caution) 2 g
Phytosterol supplement (p. 14)

HERBAL
Echinacea
Chilli (p. 39, caution)
Stinging nettle

AROMATHERAPY
Eucalyptus oil. Put 3 drops on a handkerchief and inhale.

HOMEOPATHY
Aconite for a sudden attack, often brought on by cold weather, which causes great distress and panic
Arsenicum album if the attacks tend to occur around midnight and the person seems exhausted but will not lie still, preferring to sit up or walk around
Chamomilla for attacks precipitated by emotional tension or characterized by feelings of extreme anger
Ipecacuana for attacks accompanied by nausea and a feeling that the chest is full of phlegm which cannot be expelled
Nat. sulph. for attacks brought on by wet weather, physical exercise or an infection such as bronchitis
Take 30C every 15 minutes until an improvement is felt.

ACUPRESSURE
Great Abyss (L 9). Press this point on each hand in turn for one minute every day and as soon as you feel an attack coming on. Breathe deeply as you do so.

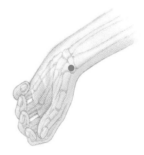 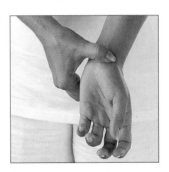

Above: *The Great Abyss (L 9) points are located in the indentation between your thumb and wrist bones.*

RELAXATION
Deep-breathing exercises and meditation should be practised regularly (these have helped some asthma sufferers dramatically).

HOUSE DUST
Most asthma sufferers are allergic to house dust (allergens produced by dust mites, cats, dogs, cockroaches and fungi). All dust-collecting objects, such as carpets, soft toys, soft furniture and feather pillows and duvets, should be removed and replaced with alternatives.

EXERCISE
Although sudden exercise can precipitate an asthma attack, regular aerobic exercise such as swimming is recommended to build up the lung capacity.

IONIZERS

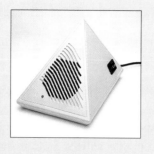

Research has shown that asthma sufferers, especially infants, can often benefit greatly from breathing negatively charged air. The negative ions produced by an ionizer cause dust and other inhaled allergens to settle. Ionizers are only really effective within a radius of 3–4 metres (3¼–4 yards) and must be kept close to the sufferer. They are recommended for treating asthma, hayfever and other respiratory conditions.

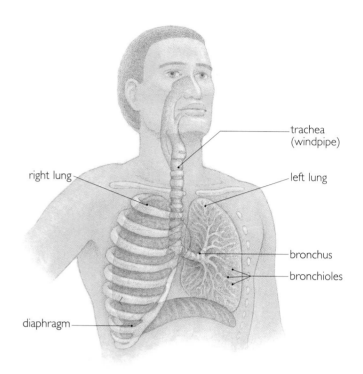

trachea (windpipe)

right lung

left lung

bronchus

bronchioles

diaphragm

Above: *Filtering processes operate within the bronchioles to keep the lungs free of pollutants and germs. High levels of contaminants, such as tobacco smoke, hinder this clearing process, leaving the lungs vulnerable to damage and infection.*

BRONCHITIS

Acute bronchitis is a condition in which the air passages become inflamed owing to an infection (viral or bacterial). It is characterized by persistent coughing, yellow/green mucus, chest pains and breathlessness.

Chronic bronchitis is more serious and can lead to permanent lung damage such as emphysema. Most cases are caused by smoking or air pollution. The inhaled irritants cause an overproduction of sticky, clogging mucus which the lungs are unable to clear. The airways become inflamed and vulnerable to repeated infection. Sufferers should stop smoking and avoid polluted environments.

DIET
Follow the guidelines for healthy eating (p. 13), taking care to avoid dairy products, refined carbohydrates and sugar, which are all associated with increased mucus production.

SUPPLEMENTS
Vitamin C 200 mg twice daily
Vitamin E (p. 26, caution) 600 IU
Zinc 15 mg
Bioflavonoid complex (p. 15) 250 mg twice daily

HERBAL
Chilli (p. 39, caution)
Garlic

EXERCISE
Carefully graded physical exercise, such as slow walking over increasing distances, is of proven value in improving lung function in chronic bronchitis sufferers.

HOT AND HEALTHY

It appears that many hot, spicy foods act as both a preventative and a treatment for bronchitis. Surveys throughout the world show that where the cuisine is hot and spicy, respiratory problems and pulmonary disease rates are low, even if smoking and environmental pollution are prevalent.

Garlic has antiviral, antibacterial, antioxidant and decongestant properties, making it an effective treatment for bronchitis.

Capsaicin, the main ingredient of chillis, stimulates the bronchial glands to release a flood of watery liquid. This loosens the mucus, making it easier to cough it up. The same reflex causes the nose and eyes to water! Capsaicin also reduces the airways' inflammatory response to irritants.

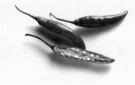

HAYFEVER/ CHRONIC ALLERGIC RHINITIS

Hayfever is a seasonal allergic reaction to certain airborne pollens. Chronic allergic rhinitis is an allergic reaction to substances present throughout the year, such as those found in house dust. Symptoms include sneezing, sore and itching throat, watering eyes and a congested, runny nose. Some people benefit from taking bee pollen. Desensitizing injections are not recommended because the results are disappointing and the treatment can be dangerous.

SUPPLEMENTS
Vitamin C 200 mg twice daily
Quercetin (bioflavonoid) 400 mg twice daily between meals (see p. 15)
Phytosterol supplement (p. 14)
HERBAL
Stinging nettle
HOMEOPATHY
Allium cepa for watering eyes and a burning, running nose
Sabadilla for attacks characterized by itchiness and spasmodic sneezing attacks
Arsenicum album for hayfever characterized by burning discharges from both the eyes and the nose (which feels stopped up) and relentless sneezing
Euphrasia for attacks which affect mainly the eyes
Take 30C of chosen remedy every 15 minutes while the attack is severe.
ACUPRESSURE
Joining the Valley (LI 4) (right). Apply firm, steady pressure in the direction of the index finger bone for one minute as often as necessary to each hand in turn.

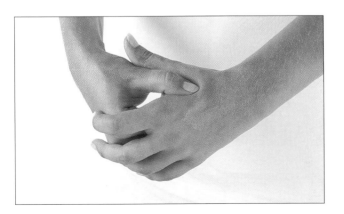

COUGHS

There is an urge to cough when the airways are infected or irritated and mucus production is increased. The root cause of the cough must be addressed for treatment to be effective. Add lemon juice and honey (p. 90, caution) to warm water for a traditional but effective linctus.
HERBAL
Liquorice (p. 40, caution). Use as a tincture for coughs caused by an irritant.
AROMATHERAPY
Eucalyptus oil. Use in a steam inhalation for coughs resulting from infection and inflammation.

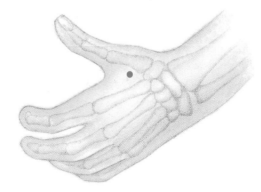

Above: *When using a steam inhalation, ensure that the towel covers your head completely to hold in the steam.*

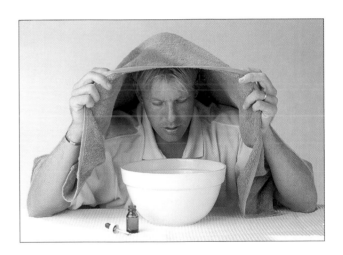

Left and above: *Pressure on the Joining the Valley (LI 4) points will help to relieve hayfever and the headaches that often accompany this uncomfortable seasonal allergy, but should be avoided if you are pregnant.*

GASTROINTESTINAL DISORDERS

COELIAC DISEASE/ GLUTEN INTOLERANCE

Coeliac disease is caused by an intolerance of gluten, a protein present in wheat, rye, oats and barley. The lining of the small bowel is damaged by an immune reaction to this protein, resulting in the malabsorption of a wide range of nutrients. In infants just weaned onto cereals, the condition manifests as diarrhoea or large, pale, offensive-smelling bowel motions, abdominal bloating, colic and poor growth. In adults it manifests as abdominal pains, bloating, alternating constipation and diarrhoea, depression, infertility and fatigue. The most recent estimates suggest that as many as 1 in every 250 people suffer from gluten intolerance.

Some children grow out of this condition and are eventually able to eat gluten. Adults who develop the above symptoms are believed to have suffered a milder, undetected form during their childhood. Approximately 20% of newly diagnosed sufferers are also lactose intolerant (p. 123). If gluten is strictly excluded, some people regain the ability to tolerate lactose.

Not all sufferers have abnormal bowel linings. Nevertheless, they still experience quite severe intestinal problems from eating gluten and are considered to have a mild form of the true coeliac disease. (Note: some people are able to tolerate gluten but are allergic to other substances in wheat.)

DIET AND SUPPLEMENTS
Excluding gluten from the diet will cure the condition in several weeks. A healthy diet and a general multi-vitamin and mineral supplement will speed up the recovery of the bowel. As many processed foods contain gluten, it is important to contact your nearest allergy awareness association to get a list of safe foods.

CONSTIPATION

Inadequate fibre intake is the most common cause of constipation, but it may also be due to a food allergy, a bowel obstruction, diverticular disease, inadequate exercise, depression, certain drugs (such as opiates, iron tablets and some antidepressants) and laxative abuse.

DIET
A diet high in wholegrains (wheat, oats and brown rice), pulses, vegetables and fruit and plenty of liquid (preferably water) is recommended for a permanent cure.

Alternatively, wheat bran is one of the most effective natural laxatives, but should not be relied upon in the long-term to top up a low-quality, fibre-deficient diet. Bran is high in phytates, which inhibit the absorption of iron, calcium, zinc and magnesium. (These phytates are broken down in the leavening process when bread is made.)

For intractable cases and people who cannot tolerate wheat, prunes (or prune juice) are very effective.

Regular servings of sour milk or live yoghurt (or an acidophilus supplement) will stimulate the peristaltic action of the bowel.

SUPPLEMENTS
Vitamin C 200 mg twice daily

Magnesium 200 mg

HERBAL
Psyllium/isphagula (*Plantago psyllium/P. ovato*) seeds as directed, or 1 heaped tbsp powder in a glass of water or juice once a day followed by an extra glass of water. Otherwise, 1 tbsp flaxseed in a large glass of warm water twice a day between meals.

EXERCISE
Regular aerobic exercise can be an effective remedy, particularly for those with a sedentary lifestyle.

DIARRHOEA

Diarrhoea is usually caused by stress, a virus or a bacterial infection. It may also be due to a food allergy. Consult a doctor if the condition persists for longer than 48 hours, as there is a risk of dehydration.

DIET
Fast for 24 hours, drinking plenty of fluids (mineral/filtered water, fresh fruit juices or herbal teas). Take regular, small doses of raw honey (p. 90, caution) and live yoghurt or sour milk (or acidophilus supplements); these have a strong antibiotic effect against a wide variety of germs known to cause diarrhoea, and yoghurt also stimulates the immune system.

HERBAL
Garlic
BACH
For diarrhoea brought on by emotional stress, choose the appropriate flower remedies to suit your personality and emotional state (pp. 64–67).
RELAXATION
Incorporate a regular relaxation routine into your lifestyle to counteract the effects of stress.

TRAVELLERS' TIP
For travellers who find themselves stuck in the middle of nowhere with a bad case of diarrhoea, mix 1 litre (1¾ pints) boiled water with 2 tsp salt and 2 tbsp sugar and sip regularly throughout the day.

FLATULENCE
Flatulence is a term used to describe the uncomfortable and often embarrassing build-up of gas or wind in the stomach or intestines. Excessive belching can be the result of the unconscious practice of swallowing air or eating too quickly. Most intestinal wind is due to an increased fermentation of food by bacteria. This can be caused by a bacterial overgrowth, inadequate digestive secretions, constipation or a food allergy.
DIET
Constipation should be treated as it is a contributory factor. The wrong sort of bacteria thrive in the digestive by-products of a low-fibre, high-saturated-fat diet, and these by-products stay in the colon for long periods of time. Follow the guidelines for healthy eating (p. 13), taking care to exclude all substances that contain caffeine. Food allergies should be identified (pp. 19–21) and dealt with.
Live yoghurt, sour milk or acidophilus supplements will restore the correct balance of intestinal bacteria and improve bowel function.
HERBAL
Garlic
Peppermint (p. 43, caution)
Fennel
Chamomile

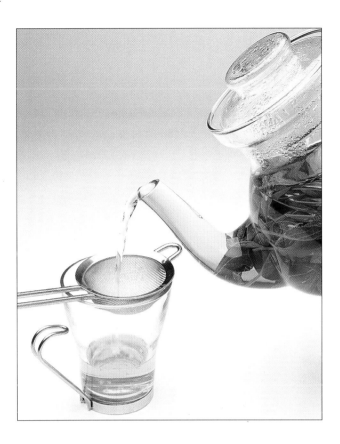

Above: *Many herbal teas and culinary herbs, including fennel, basil, chilli, caraway, dill, parsley, cinnamon, marjoram and thyme, are good digestive stimulants and will reduce flatulence caused by inadequately digested food.*

HAEMORRHOIDS/PILES
These are swollen veins in and around the anus which cause discomfort, pain and itching. Bleeding may occur, especially during the passing of a stool. Constipation is the primary cause.
DIET
Follow the recommendations for constipation.
SUPPLEMENTS
Vitamin C 200 mg twice daily
Vitamin E (p. 26, caution) 400 IU
Bioflavonoid complex (p. 15) 250 mg twice daily
HERBAL
Aloe vera (p. 36, caution)
Witch hazel (p. 40, caution). Use ointment or suppositories for bleeding piles.
AROMATHERAPY
Cypress oil. Use in hot and cold compresses to soothe and relieve painful extruding haemorrhoids.

HICCUPS

HERBAL
Ginger for recurrent hiccups
ACUPRESSURE
Wind Screen (TW 17) (below). Breathe deeply and slowly. Use your middle fingers to apply steady, firm pressure to these points for up to three minutes.

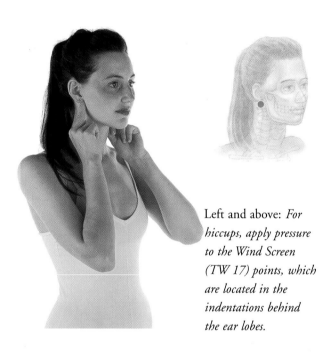

Left and above: For hiccups, apply pressure to the Wind Screen (TW 17) points, which are located in the indentations behind the ear lobes.

INDIGESTION/DYSPEPSIA

Dyspepsia encompasses the experience of upper abdominal discomfort, pain and reflux following and between meals. It can be due to overindulgence, pregnancy, exercising too soon after a meal, an excess or deficiency of gastric juices or gastritis (inflammation of the stomach lining). If the condition is severe or persistent, consult a doctor.
DIET
Exclude all refined carbohydrates and sugar. Eat plenty of fresh fruit and vegetables. Avoid caffeine-containing drinks, alcohol and cigarettes, all of which can irritate the stomach lining and increase acid production. Avoid foods which you know worsen the condition – common culprits include spicy and fatty foods. Avoid aspirin and aspirin-containing products which can irritate the stomach lining.

The following foods have frequently been indicated as allergens and should be excluded as a cause: dairy products, wheat, eggs and sugar (see p. 20).
SUPPLEMENTS
Multivitamin and mineral supplement
Vitamin C (as calcium ascorbate) 200 mg twice daily
Zinc 15 mg
HERBAL
Slippery elm
Peppermint (p. 43, caution)
HOMEOPATHY
Nux vomica if symptoms are due to overindulgence and characterized by irritability
Take 30C every 30 minutes until relief is obtained.

IRRITABLE BOWEL SYNDROME/ IBS/SPASTIC COLON

This condition is very common and occurs when the muscles lining the intestinal walls go into spasm. This causes cramping abdominal pains and bloating, flatulence (with much rumbling) and alternating diarrhoea and constipation. The syndrome is also associated with back pain and general malaise. It can be the result of one or more of the following factors: a food allergy (pp. 19–21), lactose intolerance (p. 123), constipation, stress, bacterial overgrowth or a candida infection (p. 130).
DIET
Eating a diet rich in dietary fibre can relieve IBS symptoms over a period of several months. However, as food allergy has been implicated as a cause, your condition may worsen if you increase your intake of a particular food such as wholewheat (and bran). Keep a food diary to help you pinpoint offending foods. Rotate wheat with oats and brown rice and check whether certain food combinations worsen symptoms. (Wheat, corn, dairy products, coffee, tea and citrus fruits have frequently been implicated.) Avoid substances which contain caffeine, as well as alcohol and products sweetened with sorbitol.

Regular consumption of live yoghurt or sour milk, or acidophilus supplements, will restore levels of healthy intestinal bacteria.

HERBAL
Cramp bark
Peppermint (p. 43, caution)
Chamomile
St John's wort (p. 40, caution)
HOMEOPATHY
Mag. phos. for abdominal cramps and bloating which
are relieved by rubbing, pressure and warmth
Take 30C every 30 minutes until relief is obtained.

STRESS

Stress is a contributory factor in the development of
many intestinal problems including indigestion, IBS,
ulcerative colitis and ulcers. Refer to the advice on
relaxation techniques (pp. 83–84), exercise (pp. 50–55)
and massage (p. 74–77) to help counteract the effects
of stress.

Symptoms similar to IBS, particularly in children,
may be caused by a chronic infestation of parasitic
organisms such as threadworms and giardia. This
possibility should be considered and will have to be
investigated by a medical doctor, as stool tests are
required to determine the presence of such organisms.

Below: *Some bowel problems require laboratory tests
to rule out serious infections such as threadworm.*

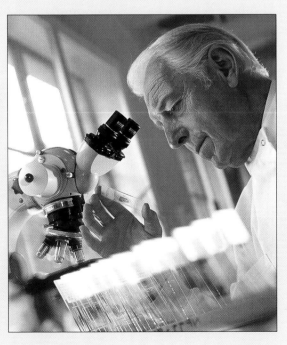

LACTOSE INTOLERANCE

A significant proportion of the world's population lacks
the ability to make lactase, an enzyme required to break
down lactose. Lactose is a sugar present in the milk of
all mammals. Everyone is born with the ability to make
lactase but roughly 50% of people lose this ability
within the first years of life, becoming biochemically
unable to tolerate milk products. This results in a range
of symptoms which may vary in severity and degree, the
most common of which are abdominal bloating,
flatulence and diarrhoea.

Note: Lactose intolerance is different to a milk
allergy, which usually involves an allergy to casein, the
milk protein.
DIET
All dairy products should be excluded from the diet,
although some people can tolerate yoghurt. A temporary form of lactose intolerance may develop after an
attack of gastroenteritis – dairy products should be
excluded until they are once again tolerated. Many
people find they can, however, tolerate fermented milk
products such as live yoghurt, soured milk and aged
cheese, as most of the lactose has been broken down
into lactic acid.

NAUSEA AND VOMITING

Nausea that is not attributable to motion or pregnancy
may be caused by many factors, such as infection, food
poisoning, migraine or an overindulgence in food and
alcohol. It may also be the result of a serious underlying
medical condition, so if it is severe or persistent then
medical advice should be sought. However, there is
relief at hand for all the other categories of nausea.
DIET
Drink plenty of liquid to prevent dehydration, but
refrain from eating food for 24–48 hours.

Once the nausea and vomiting are under control,
slowly introduce foods such as clear vegetable soup or
brown rice and steamed vegetables.
HERBAL
Ginger
Peppermint (p. 43, caution)
Chamomile

HOMEOPATHY

Cocculus for nausea brought on by motion
Arsenicum album for nausea accompanied by diarrhoea and if the person feels restless, weak and chilly
Ipecacuana for nausea when vomiting brings no relief
Nux vomica for nausea brought on by overindulgence and if the person is very irritable
Pulsatilla for nausea in sensitive, easily upset people brought on by rich, fatty foods
Take 30C of chosen remedy every 10 minutes until symptoms subside.

ACUPRESSURE

Bigger Rushing (Lv 3). Use your two middle fingers to stimulate both points together (p. 73) if the nausea is accompanied by cramps.
Inner Gate (P 6) (below). Apply deep thumb pressure for 2 minutes on each side, taking deep, relaxing breaths. (Children, particularly those who suffer from motion sickness, can be taught how to stimulate these points.) Motion bands, which stimulate these points, are also effective.

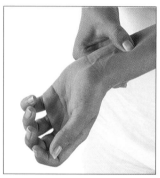
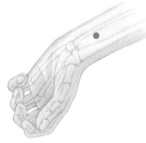

Above: *The Inner Gate (P 6) point is located on the forearm about three fingerwidths up from the wrist crease between the two tendons which can be seen when the fist is clenched.*

FIBRE IN YOUR DIET

Dietary fibre, found in unrefined plant matter, is crucial to the health of the colon and offers protection against a wide variety of diseases such as appendicitis, diverticulosis (and the infected condition of diverticulitis) and cancer of the colon.

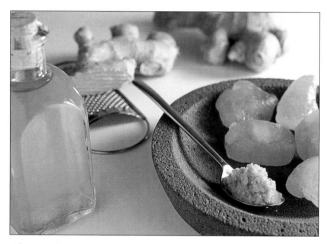

Above: *Ginger is superior to many drugs in treating nausea and is also useful in the treatment of inflammatory disorders such as ulcerative colitis.*

ULCERATIVE COLITIS/ COLITIS/INFLAMMATORY BOWEL DISEASE

This condition, which has an auto-immune component, is characterized by a chronic inflammation of the large bowel which may become severely ulcerated. The symptoms include abdominal pain and frequent bouts of diarrhoea (blood and mucus are often present in the stools). Specialized medical care is advised, but the following recommendations may help to alleviate stabilized conditions.

DIET

Food allergies, particularly to dairy products, have been strongly implicated and all dairy products should be excluded (see also p. 123). In addition, follow the guidelines for healthy eating (p. 13) and include lots of vegetables – in soups or lightly steamed. Exclude all caffeine, sugar and products sweetened with sorbitol.

SUPPLEMENTS

Multivitamin and mineral supplement
Vitamin C (calcium ascorbate) 200 mg twice daily
Zinc 15 mg
Flaxseed oil 1 tbsp, or fish oil (p. 18, caution) 2 g
Phytosterol supplement (p. 14)

HERBAL
Slippery elm
Aloe vera (p. 36, caution)
Golden seal (p. 40, caution)
RELAXATION
It is crucial to address the effects of stress through a combination of exercise, massage and relaxation.

ULCERS (STOMACH AND DUODENAL)

Recent research has proved conclusively that more than 80% of these ulcers are due to a bacterial infection (heliobacter pylori). Thus most ulcers will clear up with a specific antibiotic regime and an antacid. If you do not wish to have antibiotic treatment, the following regime may be helpful.
DIET AND SUPPLEMENTS
Follow the dietary and supplement recommendations for indigestion (p. 122) to boost the immune system.
HERBAL
Liquorice. Chew two 380 mg tablets deglycyrrhizinated liquorice three times daily between meals.

ACUPRESSURE FOR INTESTINAL COMPLAINTS

The Three Mile (St 36) point is useful for treating a wide range of intestinal problems such as constipation, indigestion, colitis and flatulence. Use your knuckles to vigorously rub these points several times a day.

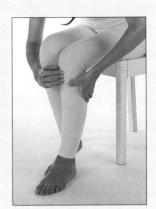

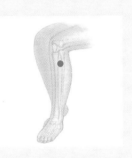

Right: *The Three Mile (St 36) point is found four fingerwidths below the kneecap and one fingerwidth to the outside of the shin bone.*

EATING FOR A HEALTHY BOWEL

The gastrointestinal tract contains a vast number of bacteria, many of which perform vital functions including keeping the growth of a range of harmful micro-organisms such as Candida in check. We have more bacterial cells in our intestines than we have cells in our body. Approximately half of our stool mass is made up of microbes. Anything that disturbs this balance (such as antibiotic treatment) is therefore associated with a wide range of gastrointestinal and health problems. Lactobacillus acidophilus, present in sour milk and yoghurt, is a beneficial intestinal bacteria which helps to keep the bowel

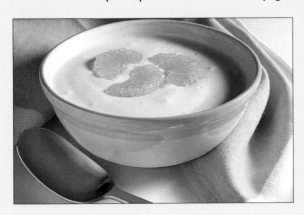

healthy and free of disease-producing micro-organisms. Acidophilus supplements contain live bacteria and, like all medication and supplements, must be used before the expiry date. (Some supplements are milk-based; if you have a milk allergy request a non-dairy version.) Take the supplements just after a light meal.

The best way to maintain a healthy balance of bowel micro-flora is to eat a predominantly vegetarian diet with plenty of live yoghurt, to manage stress levels through regular relaxation programmes and exercise and to avoid antibiotic treatment if possible.

MUSCULO-SKELETAL PROBLEMS

GENERAL ADVICE FOR INFLAMMATORY CONDITIONS

This advice pertains to all painful and inflammatory joint, muscle and tendon conditions, including all forms of arthritis, general aches and pains (rheumatism), chronic back, shoulder and neck pain, fibrositis (muscle and connective tissue inflammation) and tendonitis (inflammation of the tendons, as in tennis' elbow).

DIET

Follow the guidelines for healthy eating (p. 13), taking particular care to:

◆ reduce intake of fat, particularly animal fat, to recommended amounts;

◆ exclude artificially saturated fats such as margarine and vegetable shortening;

◆ boost intake of omega 3 fatty acids by eating oily fish, taking EPA-rich fish oil capsules (p. 18, caution) (2 g) and/or taking 1 tbsp flaxseed oil daily.

SUPPLEMENTS

Multivitamin and mineral supplement

Vitamin B complex

Vitamin C 200 mg twice daily

Vitamin E (p. 26, caution) 400 IU

Zinc 15 mg

HERBAL

The following anti-inflammatory and antioxidant herbs reduce joint pain and improve joint mobility:

Ginger

Turmeric

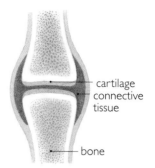

Left: *A healthy knee joint has smooth, cartilage-covered surfaces which allow full, painfree movement.*

cartilage
connective
tissue

bone

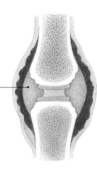

Right: *In rheumatoid arthritis, the connective tissue in the joint becomes inflamed, swollen and painful, causing deformity and restricting movement.*

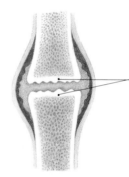

Left: *In an osteoarthritic knee joint the protective cartilage wears away until the bone ends rub together, eventually becoming worn, rough and thickened and making movement painful.*

TENS MACHINE

TENS stands for transcutaneous electrical nerve stimulation, and the TENS machine is used to control pain. This machine emits a continuous series of tingling electrical impulses into the body via several rubber pads which are taped to the skin. It is believed to work by blocking pain pathways and stimulating the production of endorphins, the body's natural painkillers. It is recommended for all kinds of arthritis, pain in labour, back pain, sports injuries, pain caused by cancer and post-surgical pain.

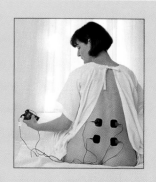

OSTEOARTHRITIS

This is a degenerative condition affecting the joints, causing pain, stiffness and deformity. Over 80% of people over the age of 50 suffer some degree of osteoarthritis. It is important to keep your weight under control if your hip, knee and ankle joints are affected. Food allergies (particularly to wheat or dairy products) may be involved, especially if the sufferer is under 40 years old, and suspected allergens should be excluded (pp. 19–21).

GENERAL
Follow the general advice for inflammatory conditions (p. 126).

SUPPLEMENTS (EXTRA)
Glucosamine sulphate 500 mg three times daily with meals (see right).

EXERCISE
Swimming (or aqua aerobics) is recommended to keep the joints mobile.

Below: *When doing aqua aerobics classes or swimming, your body is supported by the water – this helps to prevent too much strain being placed on your back and the joints in your knees, ankles and hips. Many people also find it easier to stay motivated when they exercise in a group.*

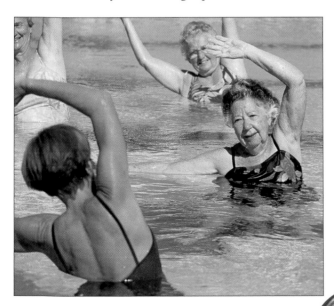

Right: *Studies have shown that copper can be absorbed through the skin and that the condition of 75% of all arthritis sufferers improves if they wear a copper bracelet.*

GLUCOSAMINE

Glucosamine, a naturally occurring compound manufactured by the body, is vital for the development of healthy cartilage. Natural production declines with age and an insufficiency is believed to a major factor in the development of osteoarthritis. Supplements help the body to repair damaged joints and should be taken for at least a month to achieve full benefits. Note that extracts of cartilage (including purified chondroitin sulphate), green-lipped mussel and sea cucumber can help osteoarthritis for similar reasons. However, they contain glucosamine in a much more complex form, which is not as easily absorbed and the results are less predictable. Some cases of rheumatoid arthritis also benefit from glucosamine supplements.

RHEUMATOID ARTHRITIS

This is a chronic inflammatory condition affecting the whole body but primarily manifesting in the joints, making them warm, tender, swollen and eventually deformed. It is an auto-immune condition in which the body attacks its own tissue, and can strike at any age.

Food allergy (to one or more foods) should be considered before anything else if the condition starts early in life. Commonly implicated allergens are wheat, corn, oats, yeast, milk, eggs, chicken, pork, coffee, tea and sugar. See pp. 19–21 for advice on exclusion diets.

GENERAL
See general advice for inflammatory conditions (p. 126).

SUPPLEMENTS (EXTRA)
Green-lipped mussel freeze-dried extract as directed. This anti-inflammatory, EPA-rich extract has been shown to help 70% of sufferers.
Digestive enzyme complex as directed
Phytosterol supplement (p. 14)

HERBAL (ADDITIONAL)
Devil's claw (p. 128)

EXERCISE
Swimming (or aqua aerobics) is recommended to keep joints mobile.

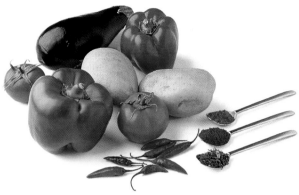

Above: *Some sufferers of rheumatoid arthritis have an allergy to the Solanum (nightshade) family – which includes potato, tomato, green and red peppers, aubergine, cayenne, paprika and tobacco – and experience total relief if these are excluded from the diet.*

GOUT

Gout is a form of arthritis, mainly affecting older men, caused by the precipitation of uric acid crystals into the joints, which become red, swollen and painful.

GENERAL

Follow the general advice for inflammatory conditions (p. 126), particularly the supplementation with vitamin C, which increases the excretion of uric acid.

DIET

Keep weight under control and exclude foods which increase uric acid levels, especially sugar, caffeine, organ meats, seafoods, pulses and yeast extracts.

SUPPLEMENTS (EXTRA)

Magnesium 300 mg

HERBAL (EXTRA)

Celery seed (p. 36, caution)

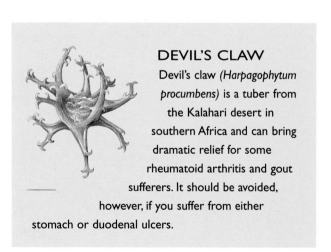

DEVIL'S CLAW

Devil's claw *(Harpagophytum procumbens)* is a tuber from the Kalahari desert in southern Africa and can bring dramatic relief for some rheumatoid arthritis and gout sufferers. It should be avoided, however, if you suffer from either stomach or duodenal ulcers.

BACK PAIN

Most cases of back pain are caused by muscle spasm (which can be extremely painful) and can lead to inflammation of the affected site. Bed rest should be the mainstay of any treatment. If the pain persists, consult a chiropractor, especially if you experience nervous system problems such as sciatica.

GENERAL

See general advice for inflammatory conditions (p. 126).

AROMATHERAPY

Chamomile, eucalyptus (p. 49, caution), lavender or rosemary oil . Use in a very cold compress for acute painful conditions. Repeat every hour until relief is obtained. Massage with 10 drops essential oil mixed with 2 tbsp carrier oil for less painful conditions.

ACUPRESSURE

Commanding Middle (B 54) (below). Stimulate these points for a minute several times an hour until pain is relieved. The best way to do this is to lie on your back, bring your knees up to your chest and place your fingertips in the centre of the knee crease. Use your arms to gently rock your knees back and forth as you maintain pressure on this point. (These points will also relieve arthritis of the back, hips and knees.)

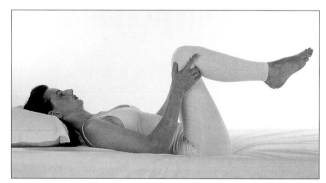

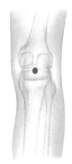

Above and right: *The Commanding Middle (B 54) points are located in the centre of the back knee creases.*

ADVICE FOR AVOIDING BACK PAIN

◆ Practise the Salute to the Sun yoga sequence (p. 55) every morning. This will give the spine suppleness and strength.
◆ Pay attention to your posture. When driving or sitting for long periods, support your lower back properly with a cushion or lumbar roll. Avoid crossing your legs, as this distorts your spine and pelvis.
◆ Ensure that your working surfaces are at the correct height so you don't slouch or hunch your shoulders.
◆ Use a firm but comfortable mattress.

◆ If you lift anything, do it with a straight back, making sure that you bend at the knees and keep the load close to your body.
◆ When carrying heavy loads, distribute them equally between both hands. Avoid always carrying a shoulder bag on the same shoulder.
◆ Avoid high-heeled shoes, as they alter the alignment of the spine.
◆ Avoid activities and sports (such as squash) which involve twisting while bending.

OSTEOPOROSIS

See p. 95.

CRAMP

This is a painful involuntary contraction of a muscle which may be due to a nutrient deficiency, poor circulation, fatigue or excessive loss of salt.
SUPPLEMENTS
Multivitamin and mineral supplement
Vitamin E (p. 26, caution) 400 IU
Calcium 500 mg twice daily
Magnesium 250 mg twice daily
HERBAL
Cramp bark
HOMEOPATHY
Cuprum for cramps in calves and feet
Mag. phos. for cramps with radiating pains which are relieved by warmth
Take 30C of chosen remedy every 10 minutes until relief is obtained.

PAIN-RELIEVING HERBS

Chamomile, eucalyptus, lavender and rosemary essential oils are pain-relieving and anti-inflammatory, and should be used during a massage or in a warm compress. Use a cold compress if the joint is acutely inflamed. Herbal ointments containing St John's wort or chilli (capsaicin) will relieve inflammation and pain.

RESTLESS LEG SYNDROME

This is a constant need to move your legs, particularly in bed.
DIET
Avoid all caffeine-containing drinks, foods (including cocoa and chocolate) and medications.
SUPPLEMENTS
Multivitamin and mineral supplement
Folic acid 1 000 mcg
Vitamin C 200 mg twice daily
Vitamin E (p. 26, caution) 400 IU

YOUR WORKING ENVIRONMENT

Long periods of repetitive motion, such as typing, coupled with an improper work environment are linked with a range of problems from repetitive strain injury to back pain. The guidelines below will help you to avoid these problems.
◆ Make sure your feet are flat on the floor.
◆ Support the small of your back.
◆ Keep your wrists straight and avoid resting them on a hard surface while working.
◆ Use a light touch when using a keyboard or mouse, or when writing.
◆ Keep your elbows level with or above your wrists.
◆ Seat yourself so that your eyes are level with the top of your computer screen.
◆ Take regular breaks and practise stretching and deep breathing exercises.

GENERAL INFECTIONS

Infections result when the body is invaded by disease-causing bacteria, viruses, fungi (including yeasts), protozoa or worms.

BOOSTING THE IMMUNE SYSTEM TO FIGHT OFF INFECTION

- For acute infections accompanied by fever, fast for 24 hours and stay in bed. Drink at least six glasses of mineral or filtered water daily.
- Eat plenty of fresh fruit and vegetables – these contain a multitude of factors which boost immunity and help fight infection.
- Avoid all refined foods, especially sugar, as these have been shown to depress immune function.
- Stop smoking and avoid alcohol and caffeine-containing drinks.
- Avoid margarine and vegetable shortening, reduce intake of animal fats (especially dairy products) and take 1 tbsp flaxseed oil daily.
- Take a multivitamin and mineral supplement and extra vitamin A (p. 26) (5 000 IU), vitamin C (200 mg twice daily) and zinc (15 mg).
- Take a bioflavonoid complex (250 mg twice daily) to help deal with the extra oxidative stress resulting from infection.
- Think positively: optimists have better immune function than pessimists!
- Deal with stress build-up, a well-known depressor of immune function, by adopting a regular relaxation activity (pp. 83–84).

CANDIDIASIS

The Candida albicans yeast is commonly present on the skin and in the mouths of healthy people. It can, however, invade the whole body when the immune system is weak or as a result of antibiotic treatment. If you experience several of the following symptoms you should suspect a chronic candida infection: fatigue, irritability, migraine, irritable bowel syndrome, history of vaginal and/or oral thrush, anal and vulval itching, fungal skin and nail infections, recurrent cystitis (with negative bacterial cultures) and joint and muscle pains. Most sufferers have food allergies, particularly to yeast and dairy products. Antibiotics, the contraceptive pill, steroids and yeast-containing vitamin pills should be avoided.

DIET

Avoid all foods which promote candida growth or exacerbate symptoms. These are sugar, white flour, foods containing yeast (such as bread, cheese, wine, beer, vinegar, unpeeled fruit, many fruit juices and yeast spreads like marmite), brewer's yeast, mushrooms and peanuts.

Eat lots of fresh green leafy vegetables, many of which contain natural antifungal agents.

Natural live yoghurt/sour milk should be taken regularly (or acidophilus supplements in the case of milk allergy).

HERBAL

Garlic

BENEFICIAL BACTERIA

Yoghurt and sour milk are fermented milk products which contain very beneficial bacteria. When established in the gut they help to control the overgrowth of fungi such as Candida albicans and other harmful micro-organisms.

GLANDULAR FEVER/ INFECTIOUS MONONUCLEOSIS

This debilitating disease, caused by a herpes virus (Epstein Barr), is characterized by extreme fatigue, fever, swollen lymph glands, sore throat and general muscular aches and pains. It is common in young people, and recovery may take several months.

GENERAL

Follow general advice for boosting immune system (left).

HERBAL

St John's wort (p. 40, caution)
Astragalus

HEPATITIS

This is an inflammation of the liver caused by a viral infection (it also may be caused by alcohol and some drugs). Hepatitis A is characterized by general malaise and jaundice. Hepatitis B is more serious as it can lead to chronic liver disease.

GENERAL

Follow the general advice for boosting the immune system (p. 130).

HERBAL

Milk thistle

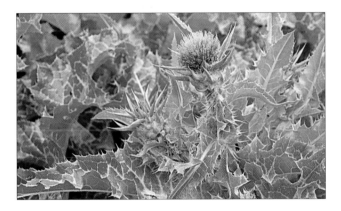

Above: *Milk thistle is a herb with a powerful protective and regenerative effect on the liver, mainly due to its high flavonoid content.*

Below: *Many foods and herbs commonly used in the kitchen have medicinal as well as culinary benefits. Raw garlic and onion have antiviral and antifungal properties. Chilli and ginger both have a powerful anti-inflammatory action.*

COLDS AND INFLUENZA (FLU)

Colds and flu are caused by a variety of viruses.

GENERAL

Follow the general advice for boosting the immune system (p. 130).

SUPPLEMENTS

Zinc gluconate lozenges 50 mg twice daily

HERBAL

Echinacea

Garlic

AROMATHERAPY

Eucalyptus oil (p. 49, caution). Use 5 drops in a bowl of boiling water as a steam inhalation three times daily.

HOMEOPATHY

Bryonia for flu characterized by a dry mouth and thirst

Gelsemium for slow onset characterized by weakness, heavy, aching muscles and much shivering

Eupatorium for flu symptoms accompanied by intensely aching bones and 'bursting' headache

Arsenicum album for colds characterized by burning, watery discharges

Baptisia for severe flu with high fever

Take 30C of chosen remedy every 30 minutes until you start to feel better.

FOODS THAT FIGHT INFECTION

Garlic, onions, apples, blueberries, cranberries, citrus fruit, figs, peaches, plums, grapes, raspberries and strawberries are all foods which help fight general infection, especially when eaten raw.

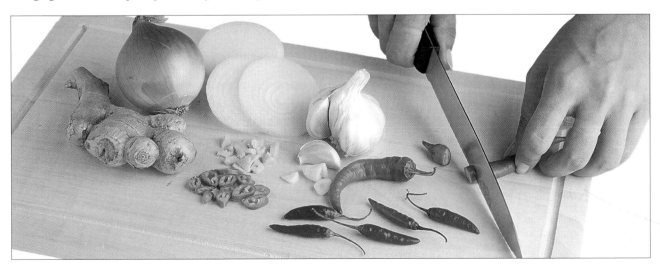

MISCELLANEOUS HEALTH PROBLEMS

ANAEMIA

This condition must be investigated and treated by a doctor as there are several types of anaemia with different reasons for their development. The most common form is due to iron deficiency. Do not attempt to self-medicate with iron supplements: these are associated with a range of side-effects and will compromise your zinc status, another commonly deficient mineral. See p. 28 for ways to increase the absorption of iron, widely present in foodstuffs.

CANCER

Diet and stress are the two most important factors to address in the treatment and prevention of cancer.

Cancerous cells are continually being produced in the body but are usually destroyed by the immune system. When the immune system is weakened it cannot cope, and cancer cells gain the upper hand. The following measures are designed to strengthen the immune system and protect the body from free radical damage (p. 23), which further weakens its defences. The recommendations apply to both the prevention and treatment of cancer, and are quite compatible with orthodox treatment.

DIET

Follow the guidelines for healthy eating (p. 13), taking special care to:

• eat plenty of fresh vegetables and fruit, wholegrains and pulses;
• reduce intake of all fats, but especially animal fats;
• take 1 tbsp flaxseed oil daily;
• avoid all salt-cured, pickled and smoked foods, especially those containing nitrites or nitrates;
• avoid browned and barbecued food, and the smoke from burning fat;
• avoid alcohol or restrict intake to fewer than 7–14 alcoholic drinks a week;
• avoid tobacco in all forms (smoking is a major cause of not only lung cancer but also cancer of the mouth, throat, oesophagus, pancreas, bladder and cervix).

SUPPLEMENTS

Multivitamin and mineral supplement

Mixed carotenoid supplement 30 mg, or freeze-dried fruit and vegetable extract 500 mg twice daily

Vitamin C 200 mg twice daily

Vitamin E (p. 26) 600 IU

Selenium 200 mcg

Bioflavonoid complex (p. 15) 250 mg. A green tea extract containing catechins should be included to protect against sun-induced skin cancers.

Phytosterol supplement (p. 14)

HERBAL

Echinacea (this should be taken to restore immune function by all people undergoing chemotherapy and radiation).

Astragalus

Green tea

Turmeric

EXERCISE

Regular aerobic exercise stimulates immune function and counteracts negative emotional states that depress immunity. It lowers the risk of bowel, breast, uterine and cervical cancers quite dramatically.

RELAXATION

Meditation and positive visualization (see pp. 80–82) offer effective ways of fundamentally altering harmful emotional habits and enhance chances of recovery.

STRESS ALERT

Prolonged stress reduces immune activity and renders the body vulnerable to diseases such as cancer. People who succumb to cancer tend to be those who bottle up their emotions. It is therefore important to adopt measures to counteract the effects of stress and negative emotional states.

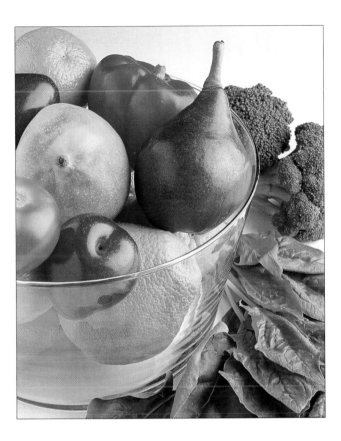

Above: *Plant foods offer the strongest protection against cancer, especially broccoli, spinach, cabbage, kale, brussels sprouts, tomatoes, carrots, pumpkin, garlic, ginger, onions, olives (including olive oil), pulses (particularly soya beans), nuts, seeds, citrus fruit, apples, grapes and berries. Fish and live yoghurt also have anti-cancer properties.*

WARNING SIGNS OF CANCER

Early detection of cancer is vital in improving chances of recovery. The following symptoms should all be investigated as they may indicate cancer:

◆ excessive fatigue and unexplained weight loss
◆ persistent indigestion and changes in bowel habits
◆ persistent hoarseness or coughing
◆ unusual bleeding or discharge
◆ lump or puckered area on the breast
◆ persistent skin sores
◆ changes such as bleeding, itching or an alteration in colour or size of a wart or mole

CHRONIC FATIGUE SYNDROME/ME

This sometimes painful condition is also known as Myalgic Encephalomyelitis (ME) and Post-Viral Syndrome. It is characterized by the development (often after an illness) of a severe and disabling fatigue which can prohibit a normal lifestyle. Although Chronic Fatigue Syndrome is self-limiting and will eventually disappear, it can last for several years and may also include one or more of the following symptoms, all of which can vary in severity: reduced mental functioning, depression and anxiety, headaches, sleep disturbances, sore throat and tender lymph nodes, frequent low-grade fevers and muscle and joint pain.

The condition is associated with a disruption of the immune system, with some aspects being overactive and others depressed. Research strongly suggests that a virus may be involved and that it can be contagious, as 'clustering' of cases does occur. However, most people in contact with sufferers do not develop the illness. Some people have gained relief after isolating and excluding certain food and chemical allergens (pp. 19–21). Candidiasis (p. 130) may also be a cause.

DIET
Follow the guidelines for healthy eating (p. 13).
Exclude suspected allergens from the diet.

SUPPLEMENTS
Multivitamin and mineral supplement
Weekly injections of vitamin B_{12} may help
Vitamin C 200 mg twice daily
Zinc 15 mg
Magnesium 200 mg
Flaxseed oil 1 tbsp, or fish oil (p. 18, caution) 2 g
Phytosterol supplement (p. 104)

HERBAL
St John's wort (p. 40, caution)
Astragalus

EXERCISE
Although physical exertion aggravates this condition, carefully graded muscle-building exercises such as weightlifting have been shown to improve symptoms, but these should be professionally supervised.

FOOD AND CHEMICAL ALLERGY
See pp. 19–21.

HANGOVER

DIET

It is important to keep hydrated, so drink plenty of water before retiring to bed. Avoid coffee, which is a diuretic and will increase your discomfort.

SUPPLEMENTS

Borage oil (p. 17, caution) 500 mg

HERBAL

Milk thistle (this herb reigns supreme as a liver restorative)

HOMEOPATHY

Nux vomica if you feel very irritable

Take 30C every 30 minutes until you feel better.

ACUPRESSURE

Joining the Valley (LI 4) (p. 73). Apply firm, steady pressure in the direction of the index finger bone for one minute as often as necessary to each hand in turn.

DIABETES

All types of diabetes are potentially serious and should be under the supervision of a medical doctor. Early signs of diabetes, which should be immediately investigated, are an unquenchable thirst, increased urination, increased appetite and weight loss. Diabetes is either due to an insufficient production of insulin (type 1 diabetes) or an inability to respond to insulin (type 2 diabetes). Insulin is needed to convert glucose into energy, and the symptoms of diabetes are due to excessive levels of glucose in the blood. High glucose levels are linked with increased oxidative stress (p. 23), believed to cause many of the complications of diabetes – such as a greater incidence of cardiovascular disease and cataracts. The recommendations suggested here are suitable for the prevention and treatment of non-insulin dependent type 2 diabetes. The recommendations can also help the other forms of diabetes, **but only under medical supervision** as this regime can dramatically reduce insulin requirements.

DIET

Although there may be an inherited predisposition, type 2 diabetes is largely caused by a diet high in refined

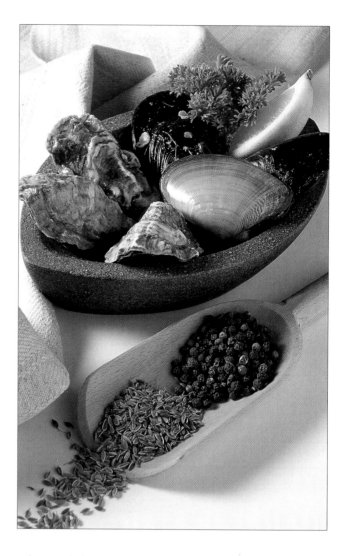

Above: *Black pepper, dill, parsley and shellfish are rich sources of vanadium, which has been discovered to mimic the action of insulin, thus allowing the cells to take up glucose.*

carbohydrates and low in fibre. It is important to make the following changes:

- Exclude all sugars including glucose, sucrose and honey. Fructose, absorbed more slowly, is allowed.
- Decrease dietary intake of fat to less than 30% of kilojoule (calorie) intake.
- Eat mainly high-fibre foods such as pulses, wholegrains, fruits and vegetables, which tend to release glucose slowly into the blood (see diagram, opposite).
- Keep your weight under control. Obesity is a high risk factor, and adequate weight loss will often cure the disease.
- Stop smoking and eliminate caffeine.

BLOOD SUGAR LEVELS

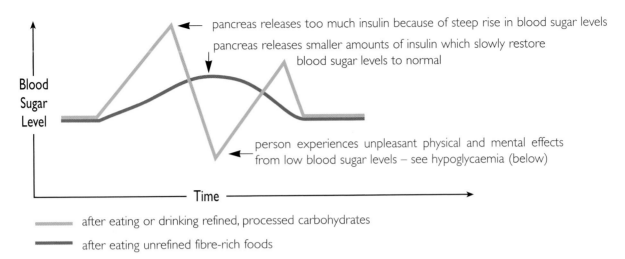

pancreas releases too much insulin because of steep rise in blood sugar levels

pancreas releases smaller amounts of insulin which slowly restore blood sugar levels to normal

person experiences unpleasant physical and mental effects from low blood sugar levels – see hypoglycaemia (below)

Blood Sugar Level

Time

after eating or drinking refined, processed carbohydrates

after eating unrefined fibre-rich foods

SUPPLEMENTS

Multivitamin and mineral supplement

Vitamin C 200 mg twice daily

Vitamin E (p. 26, caution) 400 IU

Magnesium 200 mg

Vanadium 50 mcg (in the form of vanadyl sulphate)

Bioflavonoid complex (p. 15) 250 mg twice daily

Flaxseed oil 1 tbsp

Chromium GTF 100 mcg. (GTF is known as the glucose tolerance factor and it represents a composite of chromium, vitamin B_3 and some amino acids. It improves the utilization of insulin by the cells. It occurs naturally in brewer's yeast; if taking brewer's yeast, 15–20 tablets daily are recommended.)

HERBAL

Ginseng (p. 43, caution)

EXERCISE

Regular aerobic exercise is recommended to stabilize blood sugar levels and control weight.

CONTROLLING BLOOD SUGAR

Excessive consumption of refined sugars, typical in Western diets, is associated with the development of type 2 diabetes. The diet should be regulated to include all types of pulses (soya beans, peas, kidney beans, black-eyed beans, haricot beans and so on), oatmeal, onions, apples and grapes, which are all excellent foods for regulating blood sugar levels.

HYPOGLYCAEMIA/ LOW BLOOD SUGAR

Low blood sugar levels can cause a variety of symptoms (faintness, anxiety, irritability, mood swings, insomnia, palpitations, hunger and nausea) which tend to be worse midmorning and mid-afternoon or two to four hours after eating. Hypoglycaemia is usually the result of excessive consumption of refined carbohydrates, especially sugar, although in some people alcohol may be responsible. Food allergies, especially to dairy products and wheat, should be considered as a possible cause.

DIET

Follow the guidelines for healthy eating (p. 13), and:

- exclude refined flour products and sugar (they may provide temporary relief but make the condition worse in the long term);
- eat a high-fibre diet containing lots of pulses, wholegrains, vegetables and fruit;
- eat small meals frequently;
- exclude tea and coffee, which increase insulin production and make the condition worse;
- exclude alcohol.

SUPPLEMENTS

Multivitamin and mineral supplement

Vitamin C 200 mg twice daily

Magnesium 200 mg twice daily

Chromium GTF 100 mcg (see left)

EXERCISE

Regular aerobic exercise improves blood sugar control quite dramatically.

JET LAG

If you cross more than several time zones you may experience a range of problems varying in severity from drowsy days to sleepless nights and digestive upsets. Do not take naps during the day as this just reinforces the unnatural sleep cycle. Sleep cycles are influenced by the body's production of melatonin (see p. 22). Bright natural light switches off production, making us feel wide awake, while darkness stimulates it, causing sleepiness. Use this effect to enforce a new sleeping routine.

DIET

Do not drink alcohol, and keep yourself well hydrated during the journey.

AROMATHERAPY

Rosemary oil to stimulate and refresh

Lavender or clary sage oil (p. 49, caution) to sedate and relax.

Use as a direct inhalation or add to a bath.

OBESITY

This is caused by consuming more kilojoules (calories) than the body can metabolize (use up in energy); surplus kilojoules are then stored as fat. However, people's metabolic rates vary. Some people can overeat without building up fat, while others gain weight very easily.

When the metabolic rate is increased (through, for example, exercise) stored fat and excess kilojoules are burned in a process called thermogenesis. When you go on a crash diet your metabolic rate is reduced (to protect vital areas of the body from running out of an energy supply). It actually becomes more difficult to lose weight and, more importantly, to maintain the weight loss. The process of thermogenesis is also adversely affected by certain nutritional deficiencies (such as iron and potassium) and food allergy reactions. People who are overweight and typically feel very hungry soon after a meal should consider the possibility of an allergy (pp. 19–21). Longterm lifestyle changes are recommended to reduce the problem of obesity.

DIET

Follow the guidelines for healthy eating (p. 13).

Eat plenty of fresh fruit and vegetables, pulses and oats, and reduce your salt intake so that potassium levels are increased (see p. 20). Reduce fat intake to less than 20% of total daily kilojoules (calories) and eat smaller meals.

SUPPLEMENTS

Vitamin C 200 mg twice daily. Take this with meals to increase iron absorption.

Chromium GTF 100 mcg (p. 135)

HERBAL

Green tea. Drink infusion three times daily between meals. (Caffeine stimulates the process of thermogenesis, and green tea is one of the best sources of caffeine because it comes with an array of additional health benefits.)

EXERCISE

Aerobic exercise stimulates thermogenesis for several hours after the activity and, if practised regularly, it is one of the most effective ways to lose weight. Cold showers also stimulate thermogenesis.

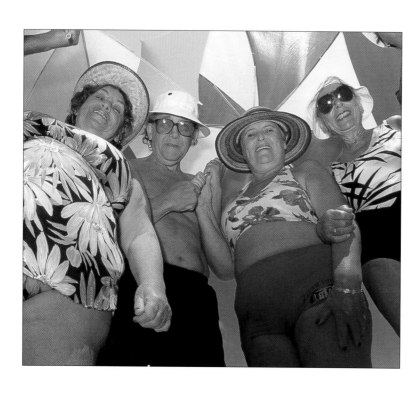

Left: *Obesity may not cause unhappiness, but it does predispose people to suffer from many different diseases including cardiovascular disease, diabetes, high blood pressure, gout, arthritis, menstrual disorders and so on. It is recommended that lifestyle changes are made to reduce the problem of obesity and improve overall health.*

FIRST AID AND EMERGENCIES

SHOCK

All accidents and emergencies induce a degree of emotional shock, which should be treated together with any injuries. Bach Rescue Remedy (2–4 drops) and homeopathic Arnica (30C), given together, should be your first line of treatment, especially if an injury has been sustained.

HOMEOPATHY

In addition to Arnica, one of the following remedies may be indicated:

Aconite if the person is panicky, fearful and frightened

Gelsemium if the person is trembling with fear

Ignatia if the person is shocked after bad news

Take 30C of chosen remedy every 10 minutes until calm.

BITES AND STINGS

Bites and stings vary in severity and nature because of the different diseases and venoms animals and insects may carry. People can become dangerously allergic to certain venoms. Severe reactions must receive medical attention immediately. Insect bites can be discouraged by applying 5 drops geranium oil mixed with 2 tbsp carrier oil to exposed skin or by using geranium oil in a vaporizer.

DOG BITES

If bitten by a dog in an area where rabies occurs, seek medical help immediately: a rabies antidote must be given within 24 hours to be effective. A tetanus booster is recommended for all serious wounds and bites from all mammals, no matter how small.

HERBAL AND AROMATHERAPY

Calendula and tea tree oil. Clean the area thoroughly with calendula tincture diluted 1:5 with warm water. Keep the wound covered with a dressing on which a few drops of tea tree oil have been sprinkled.

HOMEOPATHY

Hypericum 30C every 4 hours for the first day.

INSECT BITES AND STINGS

In the case of a bee sting, try to remove the sting and poison sac with tweezers or by scraping the skin with a blunt object. Sodium bicarbonate (made into a paste) will neutralize bee and ant poison while lemon juice or vinegar neutralizes wasp stings.

HERBAL

Witch hazel (p. 40, caution). Dab cold distilled witch hazel onto cotton wool and apply to affected area until relief is obtained.

AROMATHERAPY

Lavender or tea tree oil. Apply neat to affected area.

HOMEOPATHY

Apis if the wound is swollen, burning and stinging

Urtica urens if the wound is extremely itchy

Hypericum for all other types of painful wounds

Take 30C of chosen remedy every 30 minutes until relief is obtained.

BRUISES

People may bruise easily because of weakened capillaries or because they lack vitamin K, which is essential for the blood clotting process. Antibiotics can destroy the beneficial bacteria which live in the intestine and make vitamin K.

DIET

A daily serving of live yoghurt or sour milk, or an acidophilus supplement, will help recolonize the intestine with suitable bacteria.

SUPPLEMENTS

Vitamin C 200 mg twice daily

Bioflavonoid complex (p. 15) 250 mg twice daily

HERBAL

Witch hazel (p. 40, caution). Apply a dressing made with cold distilled witch hazel to bruised area.

Arnica (p. 36, caution). Apply Arnica cream to all bruised areas if the skin is unbroken.

HOMEOPATHY

Arnica for any painful injury

Hypericum for any injury accompanied by shooting pains (suggesting nerve damage)

Ruta for painful bone injuries such as a blow to the shin

Ledum for a black eye

Take 30C of chosen remedy three times daily (or more frequently if the pain is intense) until the bruising and pain resolve.

SPLINTERS

Remove the splinter if possible (use tweezers or a needle sterilized by boiling it for 10 minutes or heating it in the clear part of a flame), and apply tea tree oil to the affected area. If the splinter is too deep to remove, apply a poultice (see below) and keep covered.

HERBAL

Slippery elm. Make a hot paste with slippery elm powder and apply directly to the wound site. Cover and secure with a bandage. Renew the poultice every few hours until the splinter is drawn out. Chickweed ointment or raw honey can be used in a dressing, as long as the wound is kept covered.

HOMEOPATHY

Silica 30C three times daily

CUTS AND SORES

For serious wounds see surgery, p. 139.

HERBAL

Witch hazel (p. 40, caution), calendula or St John's wort. Clean wound with either distilled witch hazel or with calendula or St John's wort tincture diluted 1:10 with water. Keep pressure on the wound if bleeding is a problem.

Apply calendula ointment or raw honey and cover the wound with a dressing until healthy new tissue has formed. Do not allow it to scab over too quickly in case there is still dirt in the wound.

If the wound does scab over and become painful and inflamed, apply raw honey to it and keep it covered. Change the dressing daily and check for signs of healthy new pink tissue before leaving it uncovered.

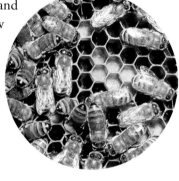

Above: *Honey is a powerful bactericide and one of the best treatments for dirty wounds.*

AROMATHERAPY

Tea tree, eucalyptus (p. 49, caution) or lavender oil. Apply 5 drops essential oil mixed with 1 tbsp carrier oil as an antiseptic dressing.

NOSEBLEEDS

Foreign bodies can cause nosebleeds, so if the sufferer is a young child, first check that this is not the cause. If nosebleeds are a regular occurrence, follow the dietary and supplement advice given for bruises (see above left).

HERBAL

Witch hazel (p. 40, caution). Dab cold, distilled witch hazel onto cotton wool and squeeze this compress over the nostrils for up to five minutes. It's best not to throw the head back or lie down as the blood may trickle down the throat and cause vomiting. Do not blow your nose once the bleeding has stopped or it may re-start.

HOMEOPATHY

Arnica if the nosebleed is the result of injury

Phosphorus if the nosebleed starts spontaneously
Take 30C of chosen remedy every 30 minutes until
bleeding stops.

BURNS AND SUNBURN

Minor burns and scalds can be treated effectively at
home. Cool the affected area by immersing it in very
cold water or applying cold, wet compresses. Do not
apply grease, butter or ice-cold water. Do not puncture
blisters or cover with fluffy fabric.

HERBAL

Witch hazel (p. 40, caution). Apply cold, distilled witch
hazel in a compress to minimize swelling and prevent
infection. Keep applying fresh cold compresses until
the pain has gone.
Aloe vera or calendula. Apply gel or cream regularly
once healing begins.
Black or green tea. Apply cool tea as a soothing antiseptic treatment.

AROMATHERAPY

Lavender oil. Regularly massage area with 5 drops essential oil to 1 tbsp carrier oil once healing has begun.

HOMEOPATHY

Arnica
Urtica urens or cantharis if there is blistering
Take 30C of chosen remedy every 30 minutes until the
pain is alleviated.

STAYING SAFE IN THE SUN

To protect against ultraviolet (UV) light damage, which
causes prematurely aged skin, solar keratosis, skin
cancer and an increased incidence of melanomas, it is
important to stay out of the sun between 9 am and 4 pm.
Follow the guidelines below if you do go into the sun.

- Use a hat with a wide brim (not a cap) to protect
  vulnerable areas like the nose, lips, ears and neck.
- Remember that water reflects UV light, so a hat or
  an umbrella is inadequate protection near water.
- Wear UV-resistant swimwear and clothing.
- Cover exposed skin with skin cream with a high UVA
  and UVB protection factor (25 and over).

SPRAINS AND STRAINS

AROMATHERAPY

Chamomile, eucalyptus, lavender or rosemary oil.
Use in a cold compress. Apply a pressure bandage for
support.

HOMEOPATHY

Arnica for bruising and shock
Rhus. tox. if the pain is worse with rest but better with
movement
Ruta for strains to tendons and joints, particularly
ankles and wrists
Take 30C of chosen remedy four times daily until relief
is obtained.

BONE FRACTURES

See surgery (below).

HOMEOPATHY

Symphytum 6C three times daily for four weeks.

SURGERY AND DENTAL WORK

DIET

Follow the basic guidelines for healthy eating (p. 13).

SUPPLEMENTS

To promote wound healing and recovery, take:
Multivitamin and mineral supplement
Betacarotene 10 mg
Vitamin B complex
Vitamin C 200 mg twice daily
Vitamin E (p. 26) 400 IU
Zinc 15 mg

HOMEOPATHY

Arnica and Hypericum
Aconite if you are extremely anxious about the forth-
coming procedure
Take 30 C of chosen remedy four times daily just before
and for several days after surgery and dental extractions.

BACH

Rescue Remedy. Take four times daily the day before
and for several days after surgery or dental work.

GLOSSARY

Acidophilus supplement A supplement containing live *Acidophilus* bacteria (*Bifidus* bacteria are often included). These 'friendly' bacteria are essential for bowel function and health.

Acute disease A disease which comes on suddenly and is of limited duration.

Adaptogen A plant substance that adapts its effects to the needs of the individual. Phytosterols, for example, may increase immune system activity in a person with an underactive immune system or bring it back to normal levels in someone with an overactive immune system.

Aerobic exercise Any exercise which raises the heart and respiration rate.

Allergen A substance which can bring about an allergic reaction.

Allergy An adverse reaction to a normally harmless substance (such as pollen, mould or a common foodstuff) which may or may not involve an immune response. Classical allergic reactions can be measured by the RAST test; tests for other types of allergies are not as reliable. Some food allergies are caused by a biochemical reaction to certain food constituents and do not involve an immune response. These are often referred to as 'food intolerances'. This distinction has become confusing, though, as it is difficult to identify the cause of the reaction. We therefore use the term 'food allergy' throughout the text to indicate any adverse reaction to food.

Amino acids The basic building blocks of protein. Essential amino acids (isoleucine, leucine, lysine, methionine, phenylalanine, threonine, tryptophan, valine and histidine for infants) need to be supplied in the diet. Non-essential amino acids can be made by the body provided the correct nutrients are present. Certain amino acid supplements can be helpful to some people, especially carnitine (for obesity, chronic fatigue and increased athletic performance), as carnitine is needed to convert stored fat to energy. Glutathione, N-acetyl cysteine and taurine possess antioxidant properties and assist detoxification. Doses of 500–1 000 mg twice daily are usually recommended.

Analgesic A pain-relieving substance.

Anti-allergic A substance that reduces hypersensitivity or allergic reactions.

Antibiotic A substance that kills bacteria. Antibiotic drugs are used to treat bacterial infections; they are ineffective against viral infections. Note that (unlike antibiotic drugs) herbal antibacterials tend to target disease-causing bacteria, leaving 'friendly' bacteria unharmed.

Antibody A protein produced by the immune system, and which neutralizes foreign proteins (such as bacteria).

Anticoagulant A substance that discourages blood platelets from sticking together and forming clots (sometimes referred to as 'blood-thinning').

Antidepressant A substance that alleviates depression.

Anti-inflammatory Substances which reduce symptoms of inflammation, for example redness, swelling and pain.

Antimicrobial Substances which are harmful to a range of micro-organisms such as bacteria, viruses, fungi and parasitic worms.

Antimutagenic Substances that neutralize mutagens. Mutagens (also known as carcinogens) are factors (such as ionizing radiation, cigarette smoke, pollution and free radicals) that can initiate cell changes, which lead to cancer. Some mutagens also promote the growth and spread of cancer. Antimutagens can help in suppressing the progression of cancer. Antioxidants also function as antimutagens.

Antioxidant Substances that deactivate free radicals and thus protect the body from their destructive effects.

Antispasmodic Substances that reduce muscle spasm and tension.

Antiviral Substances that prevent a virus from invading a cell and multiplying.

Astringent Substances that cause the contraction or toning of soft tissue (such as skin or capillaries) and the arrest of discharges from the body.

Auto-immune disorders Disorders due to the destruction of body tissues by the immune system that fails to distinguish its own cells from foreign invaders.

Bacteria Single-celled microscopic organisms that are smaller than yeasts, but larger than viruses. They can be either beneficial or harmful.

Bioflavonoid A large group of often colourful plant substances with many proven medicinal effects: they are anti-oxidant, anti-inflammatory, anti-allergic and anti-mutagenic and have wide-ranging protective and restorative effects throughout the body. They are found almost universally in plants – red and blue fruits are especially rich, as are many herbs, such as bilberry, garlic, ginkgo, ginger, ginseng, green tea, hawthorn, milk thistle, lime blossom and turmeric.

Blood brain barrier Protective membrane or covering around the brain preventing certain substances in the blood from crossing into the brain.

Carminative Substances that relieve flatulence, digestive colic and indigestion.

Carotenoid Plant substances found in red, orange and yellow fruits and vegetables, as well as leafy vegetables. Some are potent antioxidants (such as lycopene and betacarotene) and, together with a range of other carotenoids, offer protection from cancer and degenerative diseases. Some carotenoids are converted to vitamin A in the body.

Catechins Powerful antioxidant and anti-inflammatory bioflavonoids found in green tea; related in effects to proanthocyanidins.

Chronic disease A disease that persists for a long time.

Circumin A powerful antioxidant and anti-inflammatory bioflavonoid found in turmeric. It can be useful when treating inflammatory musculo-skeletal disorders and cancer.

Complex carbohydrate Polysaccharide substances that are broken down by the body to release glucose for energy. This process generally releases glucose slowly. Slow release is better for the body than the rapid absorption of glucose following the consumption of concentrated sugars.

Decongestant Substances reducing swelling and congestion in the respiratory system.

Digestive stimulant A substance that stimulates the production of gastro-intestinal secretions needed to break down food so that it can be absorbed.

Diuretic Substances that increase the flow of urine, thereby reducing fluid retention and high blood pressure.

Elemental The amount of a pure substance in a compound mixture, for example the amount of the element zinc in the compound zinc citrate.

Essential fatty acids There are two fatty acids which must be supplied in the diet: linoleic acid (omega 6) and alpha linolenic acid (omega 3). Provided the correct nutrients are available, the body can manufacture the crucial gammalinolenic acid (GLA) and eicosapentaenoic acid (EPA) from these two fatty acids respectively.

Essential oil Commercially available volatile oil extracted from plant matter, and containing a concentrated mixture of ingredients. It is highly aromatic.

Expectorant Substances that promote the expulsion of mucus from the respiratory tract.

Fats Dietary fats can be saturated (main type of animal fat), polyunsaturated (main type of vegetable fat) or artificially saturated (margarine and hydrogenated vegetable oils). The latter process generates trans fatty acids, which interfere with many metabolic processes and should therefore be avoided if possible.

Flaxseed (linseed) Seeds which are the richest known vegetable source of alphalinolenic acid, an essential and often deficient omega 3 fatty acid.

Food additives These include colourings and dyes, preservatives and flavourants. All artificial colourants (like tartrazine), sulphur-based preservatives, nitrites, artificial sweeteners and mono sodium glutamate (MSG) should be avoided. Additives like ammonium bicarbonate, fumaric acid, guar gum, lactic acid, monocalcium phosphate, monopotassium phosphate and natural colourants such as annatto are not harmful.

Free radical An unstable, highly reactive molecule of oxygen (like an hydroxide or peroxide ion) which damages (oxidizes) anything it comes into contact with – from joint structures and skin to genetic material. Free radicals are released whenever substances are burnt, ranging from normal metabolic processes to the emission of car exhaust fumes. Burnt fats and ultraviolet damage lead to many diseases, and contribute to ageing processes.

Immune stimulant Substances that boost the body's immune response to invading micro-organisms and to cancer cells.

Laxative A substance that encourages bowel motions.

Lecithin A vital component of human cell membranes. As a dietary supplement, provided it is unrefined, it is a rich source of phytosterols and choline and inositol (vitamin B-related compounds).

Liver stimulant Substances that enhance the liver's detoxifying activities and increase the production of bile (which improves digestion and the excretion of waste products and cholesterol). Liver function is also improved by limiting saturated fat intake, and ensuring adequate intakes of vitamin C and essential fatty acids.

Live yoghurt Yoghurt which contains living bacterial cultures beneficial for intestinal health (check that the label states live/AB cultures as an ingredient).

Photosensitivity An increased sensitivity of the skin to ultraviolet light.

Phytoestrogen A plant substance that helps to moderate the adverse effects of both high and low levels of oestrogen.

Phytosterols (sterols and sterolins) Plant fats that act as immune modulators, stimulating underactive areas and controlling overactive responses. A supplement should contain a mixture of sterols and sterolins (in a naturally occurring ratio of 100:1).

Protein Complex molecules made up of amino acids needed for growth, repair and maintenance of body structures.

Quercetin A bioflavonoid that inhibits the production of histamines and pro-inflammatory prostaglandins and is used to treat classic allergies. It is found in *Gingko biloba*, cabbage and onions, and can be made in the body from rutin, a bioflavonoid found in buckwheat.

Recommended Daily Allowance (RDA)/Reference Nutrient Intake (RNI) Minimum estimated amounts of vitamins and minerals needed by the human body to prevent symptoms of deficiency.

Sedative Any substance which quietens and relaxes a person and allays anxiety.

Silymarin A powerful antioxidant and anti-inflammatory bioflavonoid found in milk thistle, this specifically protects and stimulates the liver.

Tissue salt An inorganic compound essential to the growth and function of the body's cells.

Tonic A substance that helps to restore normal function.

Vasoconstrictor Substances like caffeine and nicotine that constrict (narrow) blood vessels, thus reducing blood circulation and raising blood pressure.

Vasodilator/circulation stimulant Substances that dilate (open) the blood vessels. This improves blood circulation and reduces blood pressure.

Vegan diet A diet based totally on plant foods, and excluding all animal products such as dairy produce and eggs. This can be a very healthy diet, provided it is rich in pulses, fruits and vegetables, whole grains, nuts and seeds. Soya bean protein is nutritionally equivalent in protein value to animal protein. This combination will supply more than adequate quantities of all the essential amino acids, and vitamins and minerals such as calcium (vegetables and nuts are rich sources). A supplement containing vitamin B_{12} or yeast extracts should be taken.

Vegetarian diet A diet which excludes animal flesh, but includes other animal products such as dairy produce and eggs. This is an extremely healthy basis for a diet, provided the intake of dairy products and eggs is moderate. Dairy products can contain very high levels of saturated fats, which are implicated in the development of many diseases.

Virus A micro-organism that needs to invade a host cell (of animal or plant origin) in order to multiply.

INDEX

Page numbers in **bold** indicate illustrations.